Government Is Us
2.0

Government Is Us
2.0

EDITOR
Cheryl Simrell King

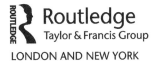

Routledge
Taylor & Francis Group
LONDON AND NEW YORK

First published 2011 by M.E. Sharpe

Published 2015 by Routledge
2 Park Square, Milton Park, Abingdon, Oxon OX14 4RN
711 Third Avenue, New York, NY 10017, USA

Routledge is an imprint of the Taylor & Francis Group, an informa business

Copyright © 2011 Taylor & Francis. All rights reserved.

No part of this book may be reprinted or reproduced or utilised in any form or by
any electronic, mechanical, or other means, now known or hereafter invented,
including photocopying and recording, or in any information storage or retrieval
system, without permission in writing from the publishers.

Notices
No responsibility is assumed by the publisher for any injury and/or damage to
persons or property as a matter of products liability, negligence or otherwise,
or from any use of operation of any methods, products, instructions or ideas
contained in the material herein.

Practitioners and researchers must always rely on their own experience and
knowledge in evaluating and using any information, methods, compounds, or
experiments described herein. In using such information or methods they should
be mindful of their own safety and the safety of others, including parties for
whom they have a professional responsibility.

Product or corporate names may be trademarks or registered trademarks, and
are used only for identification and explanation without intent to infringe.

Library of Congress Cataloging-in-Publication Data

Government is us 2.0 / edited by Cheryl Simrell King.
   p. cm.
Includes index.
ISBN 978–0-7656-2501–4 (cloth : alk. paper)—ISBN 978–0-7656-2502–1 (pbk. : alk. paper)
1. Political participation—United States. 2. Political planning—United States—Citizen
participation. 3. Bureaucracy—United States. 4. Democracy—United States.
I. King, Cheryl Simrell.

JK1764.G67 2011
320.973—dc22
                               2010044469

ISBN 13: 9780765625021 (pbk)
ISBN 13: 9780765625014 (hbk)

Contents

Preface   vii

Part I. Introduction   **1**

1. The Context: Citizens, Administrators, and Their Discontents
   Cheryl Simrell King and Renee Nank   3

2. Citizens and Administrators: The Possibilities and Dilemmas
   Cheryl Simrell King   17

Part II. Democracy and Engagement Through Different Lenses   **29**

3. Democracy as a Way of Life: Rethinking the Places and Practices
   of Public Administration
   Kelly Campbell Rawlings and Thomas Catlaw   31

4. The Citizenship Role of the Public Professional: Imagining
   Private Lives and Alternative Futures
   Richard C. Box   59

5. Cultivating and Sustaining Empathy as a Normative Value
   in Public Administration
   Lisa A. Zanetti   76

6. Models of Citizen Participation: Measuring Engagement
   and Collaboration
   Mary M. Timney   86

v

vi

7. Democratic Governance through Public-Nonprofit Partnerships: Reclaiming "A Usable Past" from the Settlement House Movement
Jennifer K. Alexander   101

Part III. Stories of Practice   **117**

8. The EPA Seeks Its Role in Communities:
Evolutionary Engagement
Walter W. Kovalick Jr., Alan Walts, and Suzanne Wells   119

9. Obituary: Team Metro
Claire Mostel   147

10. Eliminating Institutional Racism within Local Government:
The City of Seattle Race and Social Justice Initiative
Elliott Bronstein, Glenn Harris, Ron Harris-White,
and Julie Nelson   157

11. A Case of Transformational Change: Making Sustainability
Real in the City of Olympia
Michael Mucha   174

12. Think Global, Act Local? A Short Story
Larry S. Luton   185

Part IV. Imagining the Possibilities   **213**

13. Imagining the Possibilities
Cheryl Simrell King and Ryan K. Warner   215

About the Editors and Contributors   223
Index   229

Preface

*I don't know . . . there seems to be a lot of talk . . . about
reinventing citizenship, what it means. What is this group
that bombed the building in Oklahoma really saying?
. . . isn't government really us? I don't think that people
understand that . . . it affects their lives and they get to
have a say in what it does. They seem so helpless.
If only they knew how much power they had.*
—Karen Verill
President, Washington State League of Women Voters
(Frankus 1995)

Government Is Us: Public Administration in an Antigovernment Era was born
of a moment in 1995. Camilla Stivers and I were walking on the campus of
Kent State University where we visited the memorial to the students killed
and injured by the Ohio National Guard in May 1970. I had recently been to
the event commemorating the twenty-fifth anniversary, which got me thinking about whether or not citizen-government relationships had substantively
improved since 1970.

We were walking in the wake of the April 19, 1995 bombing of the Alfred
P. Murrah building in Oklahoma City, one the most significant instances of
domestic terrorism in the history of the United States. Cam's reaction to the
bombing, after the initial horror, was to try to understand how the state of
citizen-government relations could be such to engender such action. One might
dismiss the Oklahoma City bombing as the work of a madman, of one of the
ever-present people on the fringe that harbor violent feelings toward government of any sort. Yet this was more than a singular event. The bombing took
place in a period, not unlike today, of increasing antigovernment sentiment
and a sense of deep unease among government workers. And the bombing
targeted public workers, not politicians or the halls of Congress. Cam said:

viii PREFACE

> It seemed as if the sad state of government–citizen relations, which the bombing drove one to contemplate, came down finally not to theories of American government but to relationships among people, and particularly between government workers and the citizens they aim to serve. If there was something gone radically awry with citizens' perceptions of governments, perhaps one of the ways to improving their feelings was to change the quality of the interactions between the two—to make it possible for them to say, and mean, that "government is us." (King, Stivers, and Collaborators 1998, xiii)

The United States was founded on serious antigovernment sentiment, and skepticism toward government seems part of our national genetic makeup. A certain level of skepticism and intolerance toward the aggrandizing and egoism of bureaucracy is healthy; however, in 1995 it seemed citizens[1] of the United States were expressing unparalleled levels of discontent, distrust, and anger. As we've seen since, these were but the tip of the iceberg. Almost continuously since 1995, U.S. citizens' attitudes toward their governments have been steadily declining (Pew Research Center for People and the Press 2010). In response, governments seem to dig themselves deeper, further alienating and frustrating citizens.

As we were walking in 1995, Cam and I talked about the response of public administration scholars to the antigovernment vehemence of that time and recognized that the scholarly response of defending government in the face of antigovernment attacks, the tragic and the banal, was insufficient. In the field of public administration, scholars were defending the legitimacy of public administration and administrators and attempting to source that legitimacy in expertise, power, law, virtue, and leadership (Cooper 2006; Warren 1993; Spicer and Terry 1993a, 1993b; Stivers 1993; Wamsley et al. 1990; Osborne and Gaebler 1992; Rohr 1986). Cam and I felt legitimacy was not the problem. The problem wasn't that administration was seen as an illegitimate actor in the public domain. The problem, as we saw it, was that citizens weren't sufficiently connected to their governments—that we didn't see government as us (for many good, and not so good, reasons).

The key intention of our work in the first edition was to address and attempt to bridge the disconnect between citizens and their governments. We framed citizen discontent in its historical, political, and economic roots. And we presented examples of best practices and of positive relationship building between citizens and administrative agencies and processes. We believed that the time was ripe for rethinking the relationships between administration (bureaucracy), administrators (public service workers), and citizens. As Stivers (1990) said:

PREFACE   ix

> If the public service is debased in the eyes of the citizens and presidents alike, if the notion of the public interest is empty of any content save compromise, if citizens and bureaucrats no longer trust one another . . . perhaps these are reason enough to refocus the American dialogue so that citizens are included in the conversation. (253)

Engendering a more active citizenry and administration requires rethinking how we define citizen and administrator roles in both politics and administration. Our work in the original edition was based upon the belief that citizens wanted a more active role, becoming more than passive observers, consumers, or customers of public services. And we believed that public workers, both those on the firing line and those in management jobs more removed from direct service, wanted to take active steps to help remedy citizen discontent, not by papering it over with public relation efforts, but by engaging with citizens in the process of coproduction.

Government Is Us: Public Administration in an Antigovernment Era was a project of thirteen collaborators, people who had stories to tell that illuminated the issues involved in administrator–citizen collaboration. The collaboration of the first volume was purposive. The book project had to reflect what we were advocating: collaborative work that comes out of deep, full relationships. The thirteen original collaborators created something that turned out to be a rather successful project. The book was used in many classrooms and, most important, public administrators read the book and many were inspired to create more opportunities for citizen engagement in their work.

As I've written elsewhere (King 2007), transformative movements seem to happen in stages. The first stage involves *coming to consciousness*—where we recognize that transformation and change is needed—and includes calls for change that are often ideological, theoretical, and dogmatic. The questions of *why* or *whether* get answered in this first stage. The first edition of this book appeared during the first stage of the current citizen participation movement in the United States, which has been in process for more than thirty years. That stage began, more or less, with the community-based reforms of the Great Society programs, including the reforms suggested by the new public administration movement (Frederickson 1980; Marini 1971) and continuing in contemporary "citizen-centered governance" movements (see: Barber 1984; Box 1998; Frederickson 1997; Gawthrop 1998; McSwite 1997; Thomas 1995). In the last thirty years or so, public administrators and public administration scholars have become conscious of the importance of citizen involvement in administration. The first edition of this book, which reflected first wave movements, was normative and a bit dogmatic: we were sure that citizen participation and engagement was the answer to what we

x PREFACE

saw as relationship problems plaguing citizens and administrators. Our argument was surprisingly innovative (it needs to be argued over and over again and is likely to appear innovative across the ages): citizens should be involved in and with their governments. We also argued, along with others writing in this area, why it was important to do so. In addition, we supplied some stories of successful practices.

Fast-forward fifteen years from the time Cam and I walked on the Kent State campus. We, in the United States, find ourselves embroiled in a remarkably similar antigovernment era. The fifteenth anniversary of the bombing of the Alfred P. Murrah building (April 19, 2010) occurred just two months after a pilot, enraged at the federal government, flew a small plane into an Internal Revenue Service office in Austin, Texas. A month after that, the FBI conducted a series of raids, detaining members of the Hutaree Militia on criminal charges—the militia was allegedly plotting to kill law enforcement officers. According to the Southern Poverty Law Center, nationwide, the patriot/antigovernment movement has grown dramatically; the number of hate groups in the United States has increased by 54 percent since 2000, and hate groups are feeding a growing antigovernment militia movement (Southern Poverty Law Center 2010). Extremism seems to be on the rise, fueled this time by very active media outlets and the power of the Internet and social media. We've even seen a new "political party" emerge out of the extremism: the conservative, antitax/antigovernment Tea Party.

Sadly and ironically, fifteen years since the birth of the first edition of this book, relationships between citizens and their governments remain as complicated as they were in 1995, and possibly even more so. This is evidenced by extremism and the active struggle between citizens and governments throughout the United States. This struggle occurs in the wake of some very effective citizen participation/engagement movements, practices, and intentions that have been crafted over the past fifteen years. This is not to say that citizen participation/engagement practices have not had positive effects— they've had many. But the relationship problems between citizens and their governments remain.

As already mentioned, the first version of this book came out of the first stage of consciousness in transformational change movement, where the questions of *why* and *whether* are answered. In the second stage of transformative movements, consciousness is put to practice and the thorny questions of *how, who, in what, where,* and *when* come into play. At this stage, the dogmatic claims that transformation always results in positive outcomes (usually posited in the coming-to-consciousness stage) are interrogated and deconstructed. We start experimenting with the transformative practices and are quickly embroiled in the wicked conundrums that arise. In the second stage of transformation, with regard to citizen/government relationships, the normative and dogmatic claims of the first stage (e.g., the first edition of *Government Is Us*) are interrogated and deconstructed. The notion of good, productive relationships between citizens and their governments is not something that can be simply stated or obtained—things become much more complicated than they were in the first stages of consciousness.

We know that improving citizen–government relationships is not as simple as we proposed in the first edition of this book. The question of why, or whether, citizens *should* be involved in administrative governance seems to come up with less regularity—we all basically agree that citizen involvement/participation/engagement is a good thing. We also tend to agree that governance processes are generally improved with citizen involvement and that citizens *should* be involved in some way. We know that if administrators and administrative processes do not invite citizens in, then citizens will seek involvement in other ways, which are often negative. What we are not sure about, and argue about vociferously, is *how, when,* or *why* citizens should be involved (provide input), participate (be part of the process), or engage (make the plans, be part of the process and be part of the decisions, i.e., co-produce).

These are the conditions under which we developed this edition of *Government Is Us*. We don't feel we need to present the basic argument of the first edition, that citizens should be included. But we do have to wrestle with the thorny issues that have been exposed about participation and engagement in the last fifteen years. This book, therefore, is not a revision of the first book. This is, instead, a new book—written by some of the original collaborators and some new authors. We start where we left off in the first edition and expand outward. This book reflects more sophisticated analyses of citizen–government relationships; concepts are interrogated, and we are somewhat more hesitant to offer citizen engagement as a panacea for all that ails us. In addition, this edition goes beyond focusing on process change. We focus on the processes and organizational/institutional changes necessary to make governance institutions more participatory and socially just. Citizen engagement, per se, is not necessarily the only route to participatory and socially just change.

This book comes out of the same attitudes that gave us Web 2.0 and Government 2.0. Taking our cues from the online world and from recent radical innovations in governments that are based in the rapid technological change we've experienced over the last fifteen years, we call this book *Government Is Us 2.0.* We are not offering a revision or refinement of our previous work; we are, instead, offering something new that we hope will inspire positive, collaborative, democratic, socially just, citizen-based transformations in public administration theory and practice.

xii   PREFACE

The context within which this volume was created is radically different from that of the first edition, mostly because of technological change. When we wrote the first edition, the Internet was fairly new and the idea of communicating and collaborating with each other over a Listserve was attractive. Today, we all are bombarded with information and Internet-based demands on our time and energies (something that also affects the possibilities and practices of citizen engagement). As a result, there was less interaction between the authors than there was for the first edition. In addition, I came to the task of facilitating and editing this book on my own. As a result, this book is more an edited volume than a collaborative text, but the intentions and passions of the first edition remain: collaboration and co-creation are important goals and public administrators (governments) can make radical, positive change in behaviors and institutions.

I deeply appreciate and am indebted to Camilla Stivers for all the ways she shaped and influenced the first edition: her influence remains deeply embedded in this project. Thanks, also, to Cam, Richard Box, and Lisa Zanetti for the collaborative conversation that took place over the summer of 2008 and shaped this project. Harry Briggs of M.E. Sharpe deserves credit for his work in bringing this project to fruition. Our colleague, Jack Meek, got this project out of the starting gate by requesting that we update the book so he could continue using it in the classroom. Thanks, Jack, and all of our colleagues who used the first edition of the book over the years. We hope to continue to satisfy you with this new book.

My deepest gratitude goes to the participants in this project, those who were involved in the first edition—Richard Box, Joe Gray, Walt Kovalick, Renee Nank, Mary Timney, and Lisa Zanetti—and those new to this project—Jennifer Alexander, Elliott Bronstein, Tom Catlaw, Kelly Campbell Rawlings, Glenn Harris, Ron Harris-White, Larry Luton, Claire Mostel, Michael Mucha, Julie Nelson, Alan Walts, Ryan Warner, and Suzanne Wells. More gratitude goes to Richard Box (2007) because I have relied heavily on a chapter I wrote for a volume of work on democracy and public administration that he edited. Thanks to Vicki Faust, who made a significant contribution to this project through her exhaustive literature review, and to Robert Hornbein, Kiri Murakami, and Roxanne Murphy for their collaborative work on a survey of MPA students' public participation attitudes, values, and behaviors. Finally, I am grateful for my colleagues and students at The Evergreen State College who keep me on my toes and urge me to keep thinking about how we can work to improve both citizenship and administration.

Cheryl Simrell King
Olympia, Washington

Note

1. Citizens and citizenship, here and hereafter, refer to a relational view of citizenship, rather than a legal view. The legal view of citizenry defines citizens as those who have the legal rights and responsibilities afforded by the state. This definition only includes people who are legally classified as citizens. A relational definition includes anyone who resides or participates in a community, irrespective of legal status.

References

Barber, Benjamin. 1984. *Strong Democracy: Participatory Politics for a New Age.* Berkeley: University of California Press.

Box, Richard C. 1998. *Citizen Governance: Leading American Communities into the 21st Century.* Thousand Oaks, CA: Sage.

———, ed. 2007. *Democracy and Public Administration.* Armonk, NY: M.E. Sharpe.

Cooper, Terry L. 2006. *The Responsible Administrator: An Approach to Ethics for the Administrative Role.* San Francisco: Jossey-Bass.

Frankus, Sylviann. 1995. "Twenty-First Century League of Women Voters: Opportunities in New Technology, New Strategy, and the Changing Social Reality." Unpublished Master's thesis, The Evergreen State College, Olympia, Washington.

———. 1980. *New Public Administration.* Tuscaloosa, AL: University of Alabama Press.

Frederickson, H.G. 1997. *The Spirit of Public Administration.* San Francisco: Jossey-Bass.

Gawthrop, L.C. 1998. *Public Service and Democracy: Ethical Imperatives for the 21st Century.* New York: Chatham House.

King, Cheryl Simrell. 2007. "Citizens, Citizenship and Democratic Governance." In *Democracy and Public Administration,* ed. Richard C. Box. Armonk, NY: M.E. Sharpe.

King, Cheryl Simrell, Camilla Stivers, and Collaborators. 1998. *Government Is Us: Public Administration in an Anti-Government Era.* Thousand Oaks, CA: Sage.

Marini, F. 1971. *Toward a New Public Administration: The Minnowbrook Perspective.* Scranton, PA: Chandler.

McSwite, O.C. 1997. *Legitimacy in Public Administration: A Discourse Analysis.* Thousand Oaks: Sage.

Osborne, D., and T. Gaebler. 1992. *Reinventing Government: How the Entrepreneurial Spirit Is Transforming the Public Sector.* Reading, MA: Addison-Wesley.

Pew Research Center. 2010. "Distrust, Discontent, Anger and Partisan Rancor: The People and Their Government." Pew Research Center for the People and the Press. Available at http://people-press.org/report/606/trust-in-government, accessed July 23, 2010.

Rohr, John A. 1986. *To Run a Constitution: The Legitimacy of the Administrative State.* Lawrence: Kansas University Press.

Southern Poverty Law Center. 2010. "Hate and Extremism." SPLC. Available at www.splcenter.org/what-we-do/hate-and-extremism, accessed July 20, 2010.

Spicer, Michael W., and Larry D. Terry. 1993a. "Legitimacy, History, and Logic: Public Administration and the Constitution." *Public Administration Review* 53 (3): 239–46.

xiv PREFACE

———. 1993b. "Advancing the Dialogue: Legitimacy, the Founders, and the Contractarian Argument." *Public Administration Review* 53 (3): 264–7.

Stivers, Camilla. 1990. "The Public Agency as Polis: Active Citizenship in the Administrative State." *Administration & Society* 22 (1): 86–105.

———. 1993. *Gender Images in Public Administration.* Thousand Oaks, CA: Sage.

Thomas, John C. (1995). *Public Participation in Public Decisions.* San Francisco: Jossey-Bass.

Wamsley, Gary L., Robert N. Bacher, Charles T. Goodsell, Philip S. Kronenberg, John A. Rohr, Camilla M. Stivers, Orion F. White, and James F. Wolf. 1990. *Refounding Public Administration.* Thousand Oaks, CA: Sage.

Warren, Kenneth F. 1993. "We Have Debated Ad Nauseum the Legitimacy of the Administrative State—But Why?" *Public Administration Review* 53 (3): 249–54.

Part I
Introduction

The two introductory chapters contextualize citizen–government relationships in the United States and provide an overview of what we know about the efficacy and possibilities of citizen engagement. This section ends with the dilemmas before us, citizens and administrators alike, as we contemplate citizen engagement in public administration and calls for us to not forget that the normative questions of public administration need to remain front and center, no matter where we end up on the citizen engagement continuum (to engage or not to engage, that is the question). It is not just *how* we serve but *why* and *what* we serve and *who* benefits.

1

The Context

Citizens, Administrators, and Their Discontents

Cheryl Simrell King and Renee Nank

When our government is spoken of as some menacing, threatening foreign entity, it ignores the fact that in our democracy, government is us. We, the people. We, the people, hold in our hands the power to choose our leaders and change our laws, and shape our own destiny.

Government is the police officers who are protecting our communities and the servicemen and women who are defending us abroad. Government is the roads you drove in on and the speed limits that keep you safe. Government is what ensures that mines adhere to safety standards and that oil spills are cleaned up by the people who cause them. Government is this extraordinary public university—a place that's doing lifesaving research, catalyzing economic growth, and graduating students who will change the world around them in ways big and small.
—President Barack Obama
Commencement speech at the University of Michigan
May 1, 2010

Scholars, pundits, and pollsters have been talking about the state of citizen–government relationships in the United States[1] for as long as the Pew Research Center for the People and the Press (2010b) has measured, since 1958, citizens' trust in government. Each year we mark the dwindling trust in government, from an all-time high just short of 80 percent in 1958, to a low of 17 percent in October 2008 (following the financial crisis and bank bailout, matching a 1994 historic low), with numbers hovering somewhere between 20 and

3

4 CHERYL SIMRELL KING AND RENEE NANK

Box 1.1
Citizens and Citizenship

The classic definition of the politics/administration dichotomy situates the two at opposite ends of an engagement spectrum: politics is the field of citizen engagement and the place where multiple, and often conflicting, desires and needs are mediated using political processes. It is here—in the political realm—that citizenship is classically practiced, with the ideal citizen being an active shaper and player in politics. Citizens' political roles are not limited to voting, but voting is the ultimate engagement act. On the other hand, administration, according to the classic definition of the dichotomy, is the place where political aims and ends are implemented. Administration was once seen as a sterile, objective, and nonpolitical process wherein citizens had no substantive roles. However, as we know, citizens can play significant roles in administrative functions and are asking, even demanding, they be involved in administrative decisions and processes.

It is common, in contemporary conversation, to refer to subjects of government as "clients," "customers," "taxpayers," or even "the public." These terms are purposively avoided here because of the way they shift and change the relationships among and between citizens and their governments. In using the term "citizen," the intention is not to proffer a term that, by definition, excludes those who are not legal citizens. Instead, it suggests that citizenship is both a legal status and a practice.

The idea of citizenship has a long history in Western political philosophy, beginning with the city-states of ancient Greece. Within this historical framework, citizenship has long been thought of as both a status and a practice (Stivers 1990). As *status,* it connotes formal relationships between the individual and the state, including rights (voting, free speech, and freedom of association) but few, if any, responsibilities. As *practice,* citizenship entails obligation, responsibilities, and activities that make up the essence of political life, such as participation in governance and the duty to consider the general good.

---

25 percent in the summer of 2010 (Pew Research Center for the People and the Press 2010a). Poll takers' responses to questions regarding how much of the time they trust the federal government coincide remarkably with their satisfaction with the state of the nation. The trust numbers are somewhat better for state and local governments, but trust in state and local or regional governments is also at historic lows.

What is at the heart of this distrust? And whom do citizens mistrust? Elected officials and politicians or the administrative agencies and government workers that put public policies into action? As it turns out, people are angry with and distrust pretty much all of government, politicians and bureaucrats alike, and don't necessarily distinguish between the two. In the first edition of *Government Is Us,* we sourced this anger and distrust to the antigovernment rhetoric and action of the mid-1990s. Much of the antigovernment rhetoric of that time was engendered by politicians who, in campaigns, promised to take knives to the bloat of various government bureaucracies. Political party was no matter: democratic, republican, and independent candidates alike convinced citizens that governments, and therefore government workers, are parasites feeding off the resources of taxpayers. Jimmy Carter was the first president to campaign on an antigovernment platform, and most candidates for all offices have done so since. As Wamsley et al. (1990) recalls, Jimmy Carter's administration descended on Washington D.C. as a "victorious army conquering an alien city, intent on dealing bureaucracy and 'red tape' a mortal blow" (9). Both the Carter and Reagan administrations, for all their differences, represented themselves as vengeful forces intent on occupying Washington and "making the Potomac run red with the blood of slain bureaucrats" (Wamsley 1990, 9). Politicians at all levels of government have been promising to reduce the size of government since time immemorial; interestingly, it is not so easily done, and few have made lasting changes.

For our part, U.S. citizens seem to swallow, without question, the antigovernment rhetoric shoved down our throats. We neither recognize the irony that the architects of bureaucracy—those who authorize bureaucratic institutions and endeavors—are those working to tear down the edifices they designed (Wilson 1989). Nor do we seem to understand that government is us—that government workers are our spouses, relatives, neighbors, friends, and colleagues. We don't seem to connect government to essential services that make civil life possible, such as roads, sewers, schools, water, law enforcement, and so forth. We want smaller, invisible, less greedy (with our tax dollars) government until a disaster strikes or something goes wrong with services we take for granted.

Discontent in a Historical Context

Discontent, distrust, and anger directed at governments is nothing new; distrust in government seems to be written into U.S. citizens' collective genetic structure. The values upon which this nation was founded—freedom, liberty, and individual rights to name a few—go hand in hand with distrust in government. As Michael Nelson (1982) observed, the birth of the United States was

6   CHERYL SIMRELL KING AND RENEE NANK

marked as much by anger against government—the British monarchy—as by a positive desire for something new. A constitutional government may have soothed fears about governmental power, but the elitism of the authority and power structures of the government, economic inequity, the suffrage tied to economics, and the practice of slavery left simmering resentment on the part of the average citizen. This resentment took form in small rebellions, but didn't serve national ends until it became the base upon which Andrew Jackson was elected, some fifty years after the birth of the nation. Reforms enacted during Jackson's presidency (1829–1837) helped make the government legitimate in the eyes of ordinary citizens, as well as to assimilate vast numbers of immigrants during the course of the nineteenth century.

Indeed, for much of the nineteenth century, Americans exhibited relatively positive attitudes toward government. Virtually all white males became eligible to vote, and electoral turnouts soared (Marone 1990). As Alexis de Tocqueville's (1945) well-known observations attest, mid-nineteenth-century America was marked by a high level of public activity on the part of ordinary citizens. The so-called populist era (Marone 1990) of the late 1800s saw active political participation as well as active grassroots demonstrations against the federal government's failures to help farmers (Goodwyn 1978). Participation at that time reflected a very different attitude toward public life than those of the present day. Active Americans, those with the franchise, believed their actions shaped governments. According to de Tocqueville:

> However irksome an enactment may be, the citizen of the U.S. complies with it, not only because it is the work of the majority, but because it is his own, and he regards it as a contract to which he is himself a party. . . . It is the opulent classes who frequently look upon laws with suspicion. . . . The people in America obey the law, not only because it is their own work, but because it may be changed if it is harmful. (1820/1845, Vol. I, 256–257)

The twentieth century saw a significant shift in attitudes toward government. Voting rights were extended to all, although plenty of barriers kept many people from voting and from public life in general. As the nation grew, individual interests could no longer be represented directly. Instead, interest organizations represented particularized interests and pluralistic democracy/ politics was born. Governments grew as the nation grew, and these new governments were staffed by technocrats with specific expertise. Perceptions about who knew "best" shifted to government bureaus and workers. The citizenry, for the most part, allowed governments to make decisions for them, and citizens either trusted or feared those decisions, depending on the individual's socioeconomic status and race, up until Lyndon Johnson's presidency. Everything seems to have shifted during the Johnson administration. Perceptions that Johnson's War on Poverty delivered benefits to narrow groups, as well as reactions to civil rights legislation and a very unpopular war, led many to believe that the federal government not only practiced favoritism (e.g., sending working-class boys to fight while the elite avoided military service), it was also incapable of getting anything done except to waste the public's tax dollars in dubious, large-scale efforts that benefited relatively narrow groups. Thus, the citizen as taxpayer was born. In the 1970s, tax revolts took place against governments at all levels (e.g., Proposition 13 in California), reducing tax revenues almost overnight and weakening local, regional, and state government, a trend that continues in the twenty-first century. Today, as indicated earlier, people do not trust government, antitax/antigovernment sentiment is high on both sides of the political spectrum (conservatives as well as progressives), and people are seriously disconnected from or discontent with governments.

Reasons for Citizen Discontent

Citizens often have good and justifiable reasons to be discontented with their governments. Berman's (1997) arguments are as relevant today as they were when the first edition of this book was published. He argues that citizens question their relationships with government and experience a sense of discontent and disconnection under three conditions: (1) when citizens believe government is using its power against them or not helping them; (2) when citizens find policies and services to be ineffective, inefficient, or otherwise problematic; and (3) when citizens do not feel a part of government, feel ignored, or feel misunderstood by government (105–6).

Governments, however well intended, often use their power against citizens. Governments sometimes don't satisfy citizen needs and are often apparently wasteful, inefficient, and ineffective in providing basic services. Governments enter wars that aren't supported by all the citizenry, withhold information for national security, and make reforms that disenfranchise citizens or only serve a small, narrow group, thereby disenfranchising others. And, all too often, governments can't solve the sticky, difficult problems of modern life. You don't have to be an antigovernment radical to believe governments intervene too much in citizens' lives, robbing them of the basic value of individual liberty and the ability to make their own decisions about their land, families, or behaviors. Governments are regulators and jailors, and in these roles, they are often unwelcome participants in citizens' lives. Government is also mostly disconnected from citizens' everyday lives. If all is going well, government is invisible—roads are repaired, water is safe for drinking and available to

8   CHERYL SIMRELL KING AND RENEE NANK

all, the garbage is picked up, people in need are receiving food and housing, and so forth. When government is obvious, when it is connected, it is often a negative occurrence (taking a child away, telling you that you can't develop your shoreline as you like, etc.) or because something awful has happened.

For the everyday citizen of the United States, governments are the invisible, somewhat ghostlike structures that shape citizens' lives, whether they like it or not. The American Dream—in which citizens are always employed, not wanting for health care, can afford to purchase a home, live a relatively comfortable life, and have children who eventually achieve more than they have—is one of the nation's most sustaining myths. Although economic success has always been influenced by factors other than ability (privilege, race, class of origin, etc.), what nourishes our market system is the *belief* that in hard work lies the promise of opportunity, virtue, and greater wealth, regardless of economic class, race, or sex. Yet in the economies of the last thirty years, as income inequality has grown, the American Dream has become unattainable for most citizens. Poor people stay poor, rich people get richer, and the middle class shrinks as more folks slide into the ranks of the poor. Corporations gain more power and use it to influence public policy and governance. In this environment, people distrust government not only because it can't fix economic problems and bring prosperity back into their lives, but because government is perceived as an economic drain, taking away people's precious funds to support programs and practices that aren't, apparently, benefiting all citizens. In such an environment, the relationship between citizens and governments becomes an exchange relationship, mimicking a market relationship, in which citizens ask what government is giving *them* for their tax dollars and whether their tax dollars are benefiting *them* directly. Citizens become taxpayers, or customers, where money is the main source of exchange or relationship with government. Citizenship is contextualized as consumption—citizens are now taxpaying "consumers" of government services.

In this off-balance political economy, big money talks while the many voices of the citizenry seem only to whisper. And fear and consumption drive us. We live in a culture that fears the "other"; manipulating and spinning that fear keeps citizens in their place (Glassner 2000). We lock ourselves away from the things that scare us and make us feel vulnerable, often in gated communities that serve to further our isolation and separate us from others, fueling our fears instead of calming them. Terrorism has exacerbated the fear of the other; our leaders trade on this fear to garner political power.

Public policy is usually made behind closed doors; citizens are not included. Most of us are not politically active and do not participate in our communities unless we are *re-acting* to something that threatens our liberty, freedom, and security, often using citizen initiative processes in our reactionary modes. We fight among ourselves. With good intentions and for good reasons, advocacy work tends to pit activist against activist vying for the same scarce resources and attention.

Seeing citizens as customers and taxpayers and encouraging them to see themselves that way leads people to evaluate government according to what they receive. Perhaps more problematic, it also obscures aspects of public life that extend beyond who gets what—such as who decides, who participates, and the quality of relationships among and between citizens and their governments. When one's only yardstick for assessing government is how long one had to wait in line, or the size of one's own stock of government goodies in comparison to that of others, it is easy to turn individual events and allocations into a sense of isolation and discontent. Political philosophers like John Stuart Mill (1972), Alexis de Tocqueville (1945), and Jane Mansbridge (1983) argued that one of the chief benefits of direct citizen engagement with government is that ordinary people come to see how their own lives are interwoven with the lives and fortunes of others and are able to raise their sights beyond their individualistic wants and needs to something bigger that represents the good of the community. Yet for many, the notion of a public life, a "we," that is anything different from the accumulation of the many individualized and isolated "I's" seems an antiquated, romantic notion.

Administrative Response to Discontent

For the first hundred years or so in our nation's history, public administrators were few and far between. Governments were small, and their powers were limited. The radical changes of the late nineteenth and twentieth centuries, a period of time called the Progressive era, led to the birth of contemporary public administration. A need for infrastructure—public health, interstate commerce, and housing, to name a few—brought governmental agencies to fruition and created experts to run those agencies.

Woodrow Wilson's (1887) famous essay, "The Study of Administration," is emblematic of Progressive ideals. Wilson argued that administrators should be given considerable latitude in the execution of their duties, a freedom that was defensible because administration was not political (the genesis of the politics/administration dichotomy). Administrators carried out the laws, holding themselves accountable to the citizenry at large. Citizens were to serve as the ultimate source of legitimacy, not to become meddlesome, and, as a result, citizens became the source of something called public opinion.

Progressive reformers called for administrative practices based on scientific knowledge. In their view, the proper role of citizens was to inform themselves about issues and rally round the quest for efficient, expert government meth-

10   CHERYL SIMRELL KING AND RENEE NANK

ods. Progressives sought to improve public opinion by making it judicious. Citizens were assured that the experts and professional administrators were more capable of handling public problems and situations and better able to make decisions than common folk. The public service, growing rapidly due to the need for infrastructure and services, was developing into a government "of the technocrats, by the technocrats, and for the technocrats" (Kearney and Sinha 1988, 571).

Most of the growth of government in this historical period, both federal and local, was related to increased needs for public infrastructure due to significant growth and expansion of cities, the rapid expansion of the nation and dense population settling in the West, and the federal government's response to the Depression (Keynesian economics), which expanded government to stimulate the private economy. This was the historical period of Roosevelt's New Deal, and, to some extent, Johnson's Great Society. Government and the experts making it happen were seen as positive solutions to social and economic ills. This period could be considered the short-lived golden age of U.S. government. It was also the period in which most of the contemporary practices of administration—our systems, processes, and structures—were developed out of scientific studies and professional rationality/expertise and put into practice (Stivers 2000). Most of these practices are still in use today, and administrators are likely to bump up against them when trying to shift and change administrative practices to better account for the contemporary role of citizens and citizenship in the practices of public service (Denhardt and Denhardt 2003).

In the 1960s and into the 1970s, the roles of citizens and administrators in governmental affairs shifted. Growing public distrust of governmental institutions led to challenges of the legitimacy of administrative and political processes. This distrust, coupled with federal mandates requiring more public participation, opened the door for citizens to become more involved in administrative processes. However, this participatory moment was brief; it more or less expired when federally supported citizen action threatened the power base of local officials. Meaningful citizen involvement lived on here and there and in a plethora of administrative regulations aimed at getting citizen "input," usually through largely ineffective public hearings.

It was during this time that citizens became seen as clients or consumers—as passive recipients of governmental services. Requirements for citizen participation were generally treated in administrative agencies as a cost of doing business instead of as an asset to effectiveness or a responsibility worth carrying out for its own sake (Jones 1981; Mladenka 1981). At best, citizens were viewed as a constituency, the source of important political support (McNair et al. 1983) or of important values to guide policy decisions (Stewart et al. 1984). One result of this perception of citizen participation as a cost of doing business was that public participation began to be viewed negatively. It was no longer seen as enhancing administrative processes, especially when participation detracted from administrative expertise.

Treating citizens as a business cost led to a kind of citizenship that Rimmerman (2010) calls "outlaw" citizenship. As Rimmerman indicates, the failure to integrate citizens into governance processes led to "new movements of Left and Right with a strategy for promoting political, social, and economic change" (72). Both the Left and Right in these outlaw citizenship movements practice carefully choreographed "disruptive politics and potential threats to system stability" (62).

In the 1990s and beyond, outlaw citizenship movements along with environmental activism, new class social movements, neighborhood action in response to crime and other urban problems, and political organization around ideological issues led to a resurgence in public participation activity (Thomas 1995; Timney 1996) and to changes in the citizen-administrator relationship. Ironically, although participation in voting is generally at an all-time low (save the 2007 presidential vote that elected Barak Obama and may turn out to be a historical anomaly) and social and political observers are decrying a general lack of civic involvement, some citizens are demanding a place at the table in administrative decision making. Grassroots movements are on the rise, in both conservative and progressive circles, but these movements tend not to be in partnership or conjunction with governments, but, rather, in opposition. Negative citizenship (working against government instead of working with) is sometimes referred to as outlaw (Rimmerman 2010) or guerrilla citizenship (subversive and surreptitious citizenship).

When people see themselves as consumers of government services and as taxpayers, instead of citizens, there is little prompting for them to take the high road and put the public interest(s) ahead of their own private wants or to work in partnership with government. At the same time, administrators see the ideal citizen as one who understands citizenship as being a follower, supporter, and ratifier of government action, conforming to administratively defined mandates. There is little prompting for administrators to take the high road and put the public interest(s) ahead of their professional interests. Public administrators see themselves as professionals, as experts with a certain level of autonomy who are tasked with making tough decisions about getting things done in an environment of vague statutes, conflicting mandates, and an angry and discontented citizenry. Although a professionalized view of work provides dignity and boundaries to administration, it does little to encourage collaboration with citizens (especially those scary, angry citizens!). Relationships with citizens are instrumental. Citizen participation is simply a means

12   CHERYL SIMRELL KING AND RENEE NANK

to satisfy statutes, and administrators are often relieved when few show up for mandated public meetings.

Furthermore, the field of public administration has responded to calls for accountability and transparency in a managerial way, producing performance measures and audits instead of working to change relationships. Performance audits as a response to a call for accountability reflect the contemporary management orientation toward public service that is founded in the idea of the free market, where good government is government that runs like a business and creates public value (Moore 2000).

Most contemporary movements in public administration advocate for increased citizen participation or involvement in administrative governance, yet each has a significantly different definition of what this participation entails. Advocates of the new public management and collaborative public management movements view participation from a managerial perspective, building citizen participation into managerial techniques often drawn from management movements that originate in the private sector (O'Leary and Bingham 2009; Osborne and Hutchinson 2004; Popovich 1998). In these models, citizens are consumers or customers of government service and their input is important in order to deliver high performance products and services. Or, collaboration is seen as an essential component of so-called network governance, a new way of thinking about administration that is built on relationships with stakeholders and stems from privatization and contracting out movements that arose out of the early new public management movement (Osborne and Hutchinson 2004; Popovich 1998).

Through various forms, governments at all levels are seeking partnerships with a variety of organizations (private, not-for-profit, other government organizations) as a result of calls for more efficiency and less waste in government and, of late, as a result of shrinking budgets. The message here is that government can be reinvented, that is, government can be run more like a business. This has been going on since the days of Margaret Thatcher and Ronald Reagan (both often thought of as the architects of new public management, or market-based public service) but achieved something of a cult status during the Clinton administration and on the heels of Osborne and Gaebler's (1992) *Reinventing Government.* Based upon the presumption that the problem with governments is not what government does but how it works, the reinventing movement has emphasized entrepreneurialism on the part of bureaucrats, aimed toward doing more with less (Gingrich 2005). The movement takes aim at red tape, saying it is waste in government and a drag on creativity. It assumes that what people (citizens) want is not policy changes or different relationships with government, but results and productivity, an idea that is as old as Alexander Hamilton's arguments in *The Federalist Papers*

(Cooke 1961) and Frederick Taylor's scientific management ([1911] 2008). While the results of downsizing and privatization are mostly mixed (government hasn't downsized significantly, our budgets and deficits are bigger, and privatizing public goods does not make them less public), these ideas have taken hold in the field of public administration and are shaping the majority of contemporary scholarship and practices.

In the midst of all of this managerialism are active citizen movements, many of which manifest in the initiative or referendum processes. Ironically, while one may call initiatives and referenda citizen engagement or *action,* they often are more aptly described as citizen *re-action,* a more staid version of Rimmerman's "outlaw citizenship" (2010). For example, in the state of Washington and many other western states, citizens govern through initiative processes. Antigovernment movements and ideological special interests have, since the early 1990s, worked to limit the power that public officials (legislators and administrators alike) have over taxation and other resource allocation decisions. Using taxpayers as their audience, these reformers argue that government takes too much from us to fund a beast that is growing too powerful and too big. This movement speaks to a certain kind of knee-jerk citizen who falls anywhere on the ideological spectrum, from the left to the right, and engenders a sort of pocketbook citizenship where the only variable that matters is money.

As a columnist writing in the Olympia, Washington, local paper, *The Olympian,* put it: "The problem is more fundamental—'We the People' have lost control of the reins of government" (Preble 2000, 9). People do not trust their governments to make decisions that are in their best interest. While we may interpret citizens' calls as being about desiring more democratic, deliberative, and inclusive governments that drive decisions down to the people, the most prevalent response to this loss of trust and control is to talk about accountability, performance evaluation, measurement, and transparency.

There is no doubt that government needs reform with respect to efficiency, effectiveness, and citizen engagement. And there are many excellent recent movements to increase citizen involvement and engagement in government, particularly in local-level activities and alongside performance measurement efforts (Epstein et al. 2005). Still, the emphasis of the reform work being done in the fields of public administration and public policy—in scholarship and in practice—is on *how* we administer to improve accountability, efficiency, and effectiveness in our work.

In this context, are voters/taxpayers making decisions based upon appeals to their pocketbooks and to their personal frustrations? Informed decision making requires consideration of options (e.g., what are the consequences of making decision A over decision B?). Active citizenship requires being

14 CHERYL SIMRELL KING AND RENEE NANK

engaged in a process that leads to making informed decisions that have the public good in mind rather than private gain. Citizens are *participating* in governance through voting and through negative citizenship, but are usually not *engaged* in a deliberative process that informs their decisions. Citizens may be participating in governance, but are not usually *engaged* with governments in making policies and administrative decisions.

This, then, is our administrative context. If we don't engage citizens, they will practice forms of participation that stymie or limit the ability of government to do the work of the public good. If we don't engage citizens, possibilities of despot-democratic governments increase. If we don't engage citizens, we are not going to be very successful at working to ameliorate the wicked problems (Conklin 2005) of our times. Therefore, we must practice engagement—but how do we do so?

Notes

Much of this chapter is derived from Chapters 1, 2, and 4 in *Government Is Us: Public Administration in an Anti-Government Era,* co-written by Camilla Stivers, Cheryl Simrell King, and Renee Nank. In addition, we've relied upon King's chapter, "Citizens, Citizenship and Democratic Governance," from Richard Box's edited volume, *Democracy and Public Administration* (M.E. Sharpe, 2007).

1. This text is U.S. centric, and focuses mostly on the possibilities of improving citizen–government relationships in the United States. We apologize to those outside the United States—expanding the text globally is another project altogether (and we support someone doing this project!). We tip our hat to our Danish colleague Peter Bogasen, who said of the first edition something like this: "It is *Government Is U.S.,* isn't it? Not *Government Is Us?*" In his clever turn of the phrase he simply encapsulated the narcissism of U.S. scholars of governments and governance—we think our way applies everywhere. The authors of this volume do not presume to speak for places other than the United States. We practice in, and write about, where we are. We write about, and practice in, specific, situated spaces. For us, that is the United States.

References

Berman, Evan. 1997. "Dealing with Cynical Citizens." *Public Administration Review* 57 (2): 105–12.

Conklin, Jeff. 2005. *Dialogue Mapping: Building Shared Understanding of Wicked Problems.* New York: Wiley.

Cooke, Jacob, ed. 1961. *The Federalist Papers.* Middletown, CT: Wesleyan University Press.

Denhardt, Janet, and Robert Denhardt. 2003. *The New Public Service: Serving, not Steering.* Armonk, NY: M.E. Sharpe.

Epstein, Paul, Paul M. Coates, Lyle D. Wray, and David Swain. 2005. *Results That Matter: Improving Communities by Engaging Citizens, Measuring Performance and Getting Things Done.* San Francisco: Jossey-Bass.

THE CONTEXT 15

Gingrich, Newt. 2005. "From Bureaucratic Public Administration to Entrepreneurial Public Management: Getting the Government to Move at the Speed and Effectiveness of the Information Age." *Group Practices Journal* 54 (7): 11–22.

Glassner, Barry. 2000. *The Culture of Fear: Why Americans Are Afraid of the Wrong Things.* New York: Basic Books.

Goodwyn, Lawrence. 1978. *The Populist Moment.* Oxford: Oxford University Press.

Jones, Brian. 1981. "Party and Bureaucracy: The Influence of Intermediary Groups on Urban Public Service Delivery." *American Political Science Review* 75 (November): 688–700.

Kearney, Richard J., and Chandan Sinha. 1988. "Professional and Bureaucratic Responsiveness, Conflict of Compatibility." *Public Administration Review* 48 (5): 571–79.

MacNair, Ray H., Russell Caldwell, and Leonard Pollane. 1983. "Citizen Participation in Public Bureaucracies: Foul-Weather Friends." *Administration & Society* 14 (February): 507–23.

Mansbridge, Jane. 1983. *Beyond Adversary Democracy,* rev. ed. Chicago: University of Chicago Press.

Marone, James A. 1990. *The Democratic Wish, Popular Participation and the Limits of American Government.* New York: Basic Books.

Mill, J.S. 1972. *Utilitarianism, on Liberty, and Considerations on Representative Government,* ed. H.B. Acton. London: Dent/Everyman's Library.

Mladenka, Kenneth R. 1981. "Citizen Demands and Urban Services: The Distribution of Bureaucratic Response in Chicago and Houston." *American Journal of Political Science* 25 (November): 693–714.

Moore, Michael. 2000. *Creating Public Value: Strategic Management in Government.* Cambridge, MA: Harvard University Press.

Nelson, Michael A. 1982. "A Short, Ironic History of American National Bureaucracy." *Journal of Politics* 44 (3): 749–78.

O'Leary, Rosemary, and Lisa Blomgren Bingham. 2009. *The Collaborative Public Manager: New Ideas for the Twenty-first Century.* Washington, DC: Georgetown University Press.

Osborne, D., and P. Hutchinson. 2004. *The Price of Government: Getting the Results We Need in an Age of Permanent Fiscal Crisis.* New York: Basic Books.

Osborne, David, and Ted Gaebler. 1992. *Reinventing Government.* Reading, MA: Addison-Wesley.

Pew Research Center. 2010a. "Public Trust in Government: 1958–2010." Pew Research Center for the People and the Press. Available at http://people-press.org/trust/, accessed July 26, 2010.

———. 2010b. "Distrust, Discontent, Anger and Partisan Rancor: The People and Their Government." Pew Research Center for the People and the Press. April 18, 2010. Available at http://people-press.org/report/606/trust-in-government.

Popovich, Mark G. 1998. *Creating High Performance Government Organizations.* San Francisco: Jossey-Bass.

Preble, Gary. 2000. "Amendments Stripped the States of Their Influence." *The Olympian,* October 31, 9.

Rimmerman, Craig A. 2010. *The New Citizenship: Unconventional Politics, Activism, and Service.* 4th ed. Boulder, CO: Westview Press.

Stewart, Thomas R., Robert L. Dennis, and David W. Ely. 1984. "Citizen Participation and Judgment in Policy Analysis: A Case Study of Urban Air Quality Policy." *Policy Science* 17 (May): 67–87.

Stivers, Camilla. 2000. *Bureau Men, Settlement Women: Constructing Public Administration in the Progressive Era.* Lawrence: University Press of Kansas.

———. 1990. "The Public Agency as Polis: Active Citizenship in the Administrative State." *Administration & Society* 22 (1): 86–105.

Taylor, Frederick Winslow. [1911] 2008. *The Principles of Scientific Management.* Forgotten Books. Available at www.forgottenbooks.org/info/9781606801123, accessed November 15, 2010.

Thomas, John Clayton. 1995. *Public Participation in Public Decisions.* San Francisco: Jossey-Bass.

Timney, Mary M. 1996. "Overcoming NIMBY: Using Citizen Participation Effectively." Paper presented at the 57th National Conference of the American Society for Public Administration (July), Atlanta, GA.

Tocqueville, Alexis de. 1945. *Democracy in America.* 2 vols. New York: Vintage Books. Wamsley, Gary L. 1990. "Introduction." In *Refounding Public Administration,* ed. G.L. Wamsley, R.N. Bacher, C.T. Goodsell, P.S. Kronenberg, J.A. Rohr, C.M. Stivers, O.F. White, and J.F. Wolf. Thousand Oaks, CA: Sage.

Wamsley, Gary L., Robert N. Bacher, Charles T. Goodsell, Philip S. Kronenberg, John A. Rohr, Camilla M. Stivers, Orion F. White, and James F. Wolf. 1990. *Refounding Public Administration.* Thousand Oaks, CA: Sage.

Wilson, James Q. 1989. *Bureaucracy.* New York: Basic Books.

Wilson, Woodrow. 1887. "The Study of Administration." *Political Science Quarterly* 2: 197–222.

2

Citizens and Administrators

The Possibilities and Dilemmas

Cheryl Simrell King

As mentioned in the Preface, the first edition of *Government Is Us* was published at the beginning of what we might call the third wave of citizen engagement in the United States. The founding fathers never intended a participatory citizenry beyond voting. They believed that the extended geographic scope and complexity of the new American state made direct participation by citizens unworkable. Furthermore, they were acutely aware of the potentially negative effects of citizen power, restricting citizen involvement to the selection of representatives who would, as James Madison said in *The Federalist Papers,* "refine and enlarge the public views, by passing them through the medium of a chosen body of citizens, whose wisdom may best discern the true interests of their country" (Madison in Cooke 1961, 62–63).

Even with the limits on participation built into our governing processes and structures, the U.S. citizenry has been relatively participatory at different times in our history. As mentioned earlier, the first wave of citizen engagement took place during the Jackson presidency. The second wave took place during the nineteenth century and was associated with the populist movement (Goodwyn 1978). The third wave began during Lyndon Johnson's presidency. The Economic Opportunity Act of 1964, which launched the War on Poverty, called for "maximum feasible participation" by the poor in government programs aimed at solving their problems. Many of the "classics" in the area of citizen participation–engagement were written during this time, including Sherry Arnstein's (1969) "A Ladder of Citizen Participation," Robert and Mary Kweit's (1981) *Implementing Citizen Participation in a Bureaucratic Society,* and others (Crosby, Kelly, and Schaefer 1986; MacNair, Caldwell, and Pollane 1983; Van Meter 1975). The third wave was tamped down by new public management reforms and concomitant managerialism and faith in bureaucratic expertise, but resurged in the mid-1990s with contemporary

17

18   CHERYL SIMRELL KING

"citizen-centered governance" movements (Barber 1984; Box 1998; Frederickson 1997; Gawthrop 1998; King, Stivers, and Collaborators, 1998; McSwite 1997; Thomas 1995). Public administrators and public administration scholars are aware of the importance of citizen involvement in administration. Yet little agreement exists as to what this means. We tend to agree that citizens should be involved, but we cannot agree, or don't have enough knowledge to agree, about the thornier questions of *how* to do this, *in what* processes, and *where* or *when* citizens should be involved. For example, perhaps citizens should be involved in making decisions about choosing sites for waste facilities, but not in the more traditional administrative functions such as staffing and budgeting. And deeply engaging citizens in such decisions can be tricky and does not guarantee a successful result or any result at all (Berkshire 2003).

The Possibilities

There has been an explosion of citizen involvement, participation, and engagement research and practice in this third wave. Administrators are experimenting with ways of involving the citizenry, and scholars are researching and reporting on these experiments. This gives us a pretty good picture of citizen participation efforts at various levels. We know that participation is happening in governments and in nonprofits (Alexander and Nank 2009) and that nonprofits might be good places to build citizen trust and achieve democratic ends (see Chapter 7). We know the results of involvement, participation, and engagement are a mixed bag. In a U.S. Forest Service case study, Halverson (2003) found that quality participation positively affected citizen perceptions of the agency and may affect trust in government. Yet Wang and Van Wart (2007) found no link between participation and trust in government in their research. Most researchers and scholars agree that the connections between participation and trust or perception are difficult to capture empirically and that we have much more to learn before we can make significant headway in empirical research. In addition, we need access to bigger data sets that include citizen participants (most of the data sets include only administrator data) before we can fully understand the effects of participation (Yang and Holzer 2006).

For the first edition of this book, because there was so little empirical research on public administrators' perceptions of public participation, we conducted a nonscientific survey of students enrolled in Master of Public Administration (MPA) programs in selected schools across the country. The respondents told us that administering in the late 1990s was challenging given citizen discontent, budget cuts, calls for accountability and transparency, and lack of creative opportunities for doing their jobs more effectively. These public administrators said their work would benefit from three things:

improving public organizations, breaking down barriers to good governance in the bureaucratic apparatus, and improving one-on-one relationships with citizens. While respondents often felt stymied and frustrated by their jobs, they believed the possibilities for changing organizations and improving relationships with citizens made their jobs worthwhile.

A fair amount of research has been done since that time on public administrators' attitudes toward and perceptions of citizen participation. We know that participation is defined rather narrowly and what administrators view as participation efforts may be more adequately described as public relations or communications (Ebdon 2002; Wang 2001). In addition, the arenas within which participation is sought or facilitated tend to be limited. In his study of chief administrative officers in cities with populations of more than fifty thousand, Wang (2001) found that most respondents seek citizen input or communicate with citizens on processes and projects (certain functions), but only one-third agreed that citizens were involved in setting agency goals and objectives. Wang's results were validated in a later, somewhat different, study of smaller cities (Yang and Callahan 2005, 2007). Yang and Callahan found that citizen involvement is more likely to be sought in the areas of planning, parks and recreation, and public works; involvement is less likely to be sought (or to occur) in goal setting, strategic planning, and goal measurement. In addition, citizen involvement is more likely to be sought when there is significant pressure from citizens to include them (push rather than pull) and citizens are sought for input, but rarely in strategic decision making.

Administrator attitudes about participation have also been the subject of research and scholarship, and the results show mixed feelings (Yang and Callahan 2007; Bryer 2007; Yang 2005, 2006; Alkadry 2003; Brewer 2003). We know that administrators' attitudes toward a participatory ethic or way of being are extremely important, as are organizational possibilities or constraints. This research validates King, Feltey, and Susel's (1998) theory that it's not enough to engender an active citizenry; we must also engender (and educate for) positive attitudes toward participation among administrators and work to make our organizational structures and processes amenable to the participation of citizens and others.

For this book, we conducted a survey of MPA students in thirty-four programs across the country.[1] Twenty-three programs agreed to participate, and 711 students responded to the survey. A bit more than half of our respondents (370) were currently working in public administration, the majority for five years or less, and most were working in relatively low-level positions. The majority of the respondents were between the ages of twenty-five and forty.

We were quite surprised with the responses to the survey. Because the sample was not random, we can't say whether the responses reflect a response

20   CHERYL SIMRELL KING

bias—only those positively disposed toward public participation chose to participate in this survey about public participation—or if they reflect a changing tide in public administration. Yet, even so, the level of commitment to public participation among this group is striking.

Overwhelmingly, the respondents agreed (94 percent) that public participation is an important part of good governance and government organizations should do more to encourage public participation (79 percent). A majority of respondents also agreed that public administrators should be facilitators of public participation (78 percent) and indicated that public participation is important to them on a personal level (85 percent). Though still a majority, a smaller percentage of respondents see themselves as facilitators of public participation (65 percent) and believe it is, or will be, their responsibility to help motivate citizens to become engaged (63 percent). Sixty-two percent somewhat or strongly agree that they have the skills to engage citizens or they will have them when they've completed their degrees. Finally, the majority of respondents (75 percent) indicated they would like to learn more about public participation.

Some respondents told us that they believe it is the responsibility of administrators to facilitate citizen participation and they are worried about the barriers to participation, both organizational and attitudinal, that already exist. As one respondent said:

> I am concerned that public agencies interpret low attendance at meetings as disinterest and then invited the public less and try fewer creative outreach strategies. In fact, as public administrators we need to take on the challenge and ask what are the barriers to participation?

Some respondents voiced concerns about participation being limited to the middle and upper classes, and not accessible to people with less money and education. Still others don't think that it is the role of the "dispassionate" administrator to encourage and enable public participation, even if they believe participation is a good thing as exemplified by this sample quote:

> While I think public participation is present in a vibrant democracy, I do not think it is the public administrator's duty to encourage and facilitate participation. It is incumbent on citizens to organize themselves and seek out elected officials and public administrators to intervene in community issues.

And, as evidenced in the research (e.g., Irvin and Stansbury 2004, see Chapter 4 for more), some respondents think that public participation isn't always vital to the work of administrators:

Public participation is important in some cases and not in others. Many times the public does not have the skills, background, or education to make informed decisions about administration of the government. Conversely, in some cases, local government for example, knowing the desires of the public is vital.

Finally, respondents wanted to broaden the conversation and take the responsibility for participation beyond administration:

I do not think it is solely the responsibility of public administrators to facilitate public participation. This needs to occur within the education environment. We are not being taught how to engage in public discourse nor the value of participatory democracy in secondary or tertiary school. People too often surround themselves with like-minded people and this is also aggravated by the ageism in our society. People do not know how to hear other opinions outside of their own and to take the time and consideration to attempt to understand alternative viewpoints.

Respondents also identified barriers to public participation and the challenges public administrators face in trying to facilitate public participation. Barriers identified were citizens, organizations, and public administration education. Citizens were identified as the primary obstacle. Respondents cited citizen apathy and lack of knowledge about issues, public participation, agency jurisdiction, and government processes as key factors. Respondents found uneducated citizens to be frustrating participants. Other important factors identified were citizens' use of public participation to promote special interest agendas, citizens' inability to agree, and citizens' tendency to participate only when they have problems or concerns to address. Respondents wrote that public participation can be one-sided and the process can be derailed by a vocal minority. Distrust was also cited, as one respondent poignantly wrote:

Our town leaders go out of their way to engage the public and because half of our community is retired, there is a lot of participation. The barriers happen because no matter what we communicate, they continue to distrust government and spread false information, even after being informed of the truth. They think we're lying.

Organizational barriers include lack of time, insufficient funding, and public administrators' having more important work priorities. In addition, responses to the open-ended questions indicated some level of antipathy among seated public administrators toward public participation. Responses included, "upper management views public participation as an impediment

22   CHERYL SIMRELL KING

to decision making," "administration is reluctant to engage participation and claims time pressures as justification for making unilateral decisions," and "the majority of barriers [are related to] specific individual staff and their lack of public administration principals and practices." Finally, respondents indicated that public administration education is not, necessarily, providing the skills and abilities they need to be good facilitators of public participation and to manage these processes while also managing all the other things they are called upon to do.

Interestingly, we tested for significant differences in responses with regard to age, sex, political ideology, and organizational hierarchy and found no significant differences. Whether respondents were Generation Xers or Baby Boomers, liberal, or conservative they responded similarly about public participation. It also didn't matter if they worked at the lower levels of public service or were in leadership positions. Results from men and women were also similar. Some effort was made to ensure that the schools asked to participate represented a spectrum of differences along key variables (geography, prominent political ideology), and we ended up with large enough sub samples to test for statistical significance. While we can't say with assurance that the results represent all MPA students in the United States, we do have a fairly diverse sample that represents the plurality of perspectives that will make up the future of public administration.

While these results are good news when it comes to basic commitments to participation, they point to the not-surprising frustration on the part of both administrators and citizens when it comes to citizen engagement. Citizens believe the information they receive is managed, controlled, and manipulated in order to limit their capacity to participate. Citizens see the techniques of participation (public hearings, surveys, focus groups) as designed, at best, to generate input and, at worst, to keep citizens on the outside of the governance process (Innes and Booher 2004). Citizens are particularly sensitive to vacuous or false participation efforts that ask for, and then discount, public input. Such inauthentic processes simply lead to greater tension between administrators and citizens. It is better not to work with citizens at all than to work with them under false and purely instrumental pretenses (King, Feltey, and Susel 1998).

Administrators, for their part, know that citizen involvement is desirable but are at best, "ambivalent about public involvement or, at worst, they find it problematic" (King, Feltey, and Susel 1998, 319). Citizen participation is time-consuming, costly, and a burden—it gets in the way of doing one's work! Administrators are not necessarily trained or socialized to be good facilitators of participation and engagement, and, while our schools of public administration are doing more to teach about participatory methods and processes, most administrators don't feel competent to facilitate participatory processes. Indeed, there is an inherent conflict between the values of citizen participation and engagement and the structure and processes of bureaucratic government, creating significant obstacles for meaningful citizen engagement with government (Callahan 2002) and no end of trouble for administrators who have good intentions about direct participation. We are, after all, a representative democracy, not a direct democracy. And participatory or engagement efforts do not necessarily guarantee positive results or any results at all (Berkshire 2003); sometimes they simply make a messy situation even messier.

The Dilemmas

These, then, are the dilemmas we face as we move toward more participatory administrative governance processes. We know a more engaged citizenry serves government and governance. We agree that citizen engagement is a good thing and that it yields good results (Roberts 2004; Kweit and Kweit 2004; Lukensmeyer and Brigham 2002). But we cannot agree upon what participation and engagement mean or what they look like at various levels of government. For some, citizens provide managerial input; for others, citizen involvement means completely redesigning administrative and managerial processes so that engagement is an essential part of them. Furthermore, as we experiment more with participatory, engagement, and deliberative practices, more of dilemmas and thorny problems are exposed.

Engaged citizenship requires citizenship that is viewed as a status as well as a practice. Citizenship as practice emphasizes "freedom to." That is, engaged citizens have the potential to make public decisions based on their sense of the public interest, using phronesis, or practical wisdom, and experiential knowledge relevant to the circumstances. Furthermore, by joining together in civil and political organized activity, citizens may come to value collaboration as opposed to agreement. As Benjamin Barber suggests, through "strong democratic talk," which may often involve disagreement, citizens can become "capable of genuinely public thinking and political judgment and thus are able to envision a common future in terms of genuinely common goals" (1984, 197). Barber explains further:

> [It is] a dynamic relationship among strangers who are transformed into neighbors, whose commonality derives from expanding consciousness rather than geographical proximity. Because the sharp distinction that separates government and citizenry in representative systems is missing, the civic bond under strong democracy is neither vertical nor lateral but circular and dialectical. Individuals become involved in government by participating

24   CHERYL SIMRELL KING

> in the common institutions of self-government and become involved with one another by virtue of their common engagement in politics. They are united by the ties of common activity and common consciousness—ties that are willed rather than given by blood or heritage or prior consensus on beliefs and that thus depend for their preservation and growth on constant commitment and ongoing political activity. (223)

An example of this is the "Listen to the City" project, designed and facilitated by the nonprofit organization America*Speaks* (www.americaspeaks. org/; see Chapter 6), where 4,300 people came together in an electronic town meeting format to review and respond to proposals for the reconstruction of the World Trade Center site (Lukensmeyer and Brigham 2002). *New York Daily News* columnist Pete Hamill (cited in Lukensmeyer and Brigham 2002) speaks to the power of deliberative processes: "because the process was an exercise in democracy, not demagoguery, no bellowing idiots grabbed the microphones to perform for the cameras. . . . In this room, 'I' had given way to 'we'" (366).

Moving toward engaged citizenship requires that we, as administrators, think about citizen participation and involvement in new ways. This is not an easy task. To quote the great philosopher Pogo, "we have met the enemy and it is us." Much of what is required to move to administrative models that create and encourage citizen engagement is related to the "who" that we bring to our administrative work and how we practice administration. If we want a different relationship between citizens and governments—if we want or have to practice some form of democratic governance—we must do things differently and we must be different kinds of administrators.

Practicing more democratic administration, shaped by an engaged citizenry, is no small challenge. While it is relatively easy to acquire citizen input on policies and projects, particularly at the local level, it is quite another thing to engender an engaged citizenry and to incorporate citizen engagement into developing a mission and setting goals. To do so is to further challenge the politics–administration dichotomy. The founding fathers purposively set in place a system of checks and balances and left the policy decisions in the hands of representatives. "Extra-formal democracy" (Bogasen, Kensen, and Miller 2004), which takes place outside of the formal representative democratic system, was not a part of the founding models of governance and government. Administrators, many of whom are protected under civil service laws and regulations, are not elected to their positions and are not considered to be representatives of the will of the people—why should we give administrators the power to encourage, shape, and facilitate citizen power? And why should we give a select group of citizens, those who can or choose to be involved, the power to influence policy and programs for all citizens? As we do more participation and engagement work, we may be experiencing fewer NIMBY (Not In My Backyard) movements, but we are also are seeing and experiencing the ways in which bureaucratic norms, rules, and regulations constrain and limit participation and engagement. Yet, as Kweit and Kweit (2004) have said:

> Although the reliance on the bureaucratic norms of expertise, efficiency and rules and regulations may produce good policy as judged by technical criteria, it may not result in policy that citizens evaluate as good. . . . Although it may be contrary to bureaucratic norms and may appear to impede service delivery, citizens beliefs about participation can contribute to citizens' perceptions of governmental performance. The lesson for officials, generally and not just after disasters, is that citizens must feel that they are involved, for it is the citizens who ultimately determine what makes up good policy. (369)

The dilemmas of citizen participation and engagement (see Roberts 2004 for a more detailed discussion) need to be worked through. Because the intersection of the roles and responsibilities of citizens and their governments will always create wicked situations, every context will call for a different kind of "fix." Administrators are increasingly required to manage less and serve and facilitate the public good more, resurrecting the idea of public service (Denhardt and Denhardt 2003). Success will depend on a tool chest of skills and techniques that are currently being developed. Public administrators will have to be trained, educated, and socialized differently (Yang and Callahan 2005; Forester 2010). Most importantly, we must avoid focusing too narrowly on tools and techniques and keep our eyes on the normative questions involved in our work—it is not just *how* we serve but *why* and *what* we serve and *who* benefits.

Notes

Much of this chapter is derived from "Citizens, Citizenship and Democratic Governance," in Richard Box, ed., *Democracy and Public Administration* (M.E. Sharpe 2007).

1. Much of the work to support this research was performed by Robert Hornbein, Kiri Murakami, and Roxanne Murphy, MPA students at The Evergreen State College who were enrolled in the research series of classes and working on their Capstone projects. Their analysis of the data shaped the discussion here, and some of the information that follows is sourced from their research papers.

26   CHERYL SIMRELL KING

References

Alexander, Jennifer, and Renee Nank. 2009. "Public–Nonprofit Partnerships: Realizing the New Public Service." *Administration & Society* 41 (3): 364–86.

Alkadry, Mohamad. 2003. "Deliberative Discourse between Citizens and Administrators: If Citizens Talk, Will Administrators Listen?" *Administration and Society* 35 (2): 184–209.

Barber, Benjamin. 1984. *Strong Democracy: Participatory Politics for a New Age.* Berkeley: University of California Press.

Berkshire, Michael. 2003. "In Search of a New Landfill Site." In *Story and Sustainability: Planning, Practice and Possibility in American Cities,* ed. B. Eckstein and J.A. Throgmorton. Cambridge, MA: MIT Press.

Bogason, Peter, Sandra Kensen, and Hugh Miller. 2004. "Introduction: Extra-Formal Democracy. In *Tampering with Traditions: The Unrealized Authority of Democratic Agency,* ed. P. Bogason, S. Kensen, and H. Miller. Landham, MD: Lexington Books.

Box, Richard C. 1998. *Citizen Governance: Leading American Communities into the 21st Century.* Thousand Oaks, CA: Sage.

Brewer, Gene A. 2003. "Building Social Capital: Civic Attitudes and Behavior of Public Servants. *Journal of Public Administration Research and Theory* 13 (1): 5–26.

Bryer, Thomas A. 2007. "Toward a Relevant Agenda for a Responsive Public Administration." *Journal of Public Administration Research and Theory* 17 (3): 479–500.

Callahan, Kathe. 2002. "The Utilization and Effectiveness of Citizen Advisory Committees in the Budget Process of Local Governments." *Journal of Public Budgeting, Accounting and Financial Management* 14 (2): 295–319.

Cooke, Jacob, ed. 1961. *The Federalist Papers.* Middletown, CT: Wesleyan University Press.

Crosby, Ned, Janet M. Kelly, and Paul Schaefer. 1986. "Citizen Panels: A New Approach to Citizen Participation." *Public Administration Review* 46: 170–78.

Denhardt, Janet, and Robert Denhardt. 2003. *The New Public Service: Serving, not Steering.* Armonk, NY: M.E. Sharpe.

Ebdon, Carol. 2002. "Beyond Public Hearing: Citizen Participation in the Local Government Budget Process." *Journal of Public Budgeting, Accounting and Financial Management* 14 (2): 273–94.

Forester, John. 2010. *Dealing with Differences: Dramas of Mediating Public Disputes.* New York: Oxford University Press.

Frederickson, H. George. 1997. *The Spirit of Public Administration.* San Francisco: Jossey-Bass.

Gawthrop, Louis. C. 1998. *Public Service and Democracy: Ethical Imperatives for the 21st Century.* New York: Chatham House.

Goodwyn, Lawrence. 1978. *The Populist Moment.* Oxford: Oxford University Press.

Halverson, Kathleen. 2003. "Assessing the Effects of Public Participation." *Public Administration Review* 63 (5): 535–43.

Innes, J.E., and D.E. Booher. 2004. "Reframing Public Administration: Strategies for the 21st Century." *Planning Theory and Practice* 5 (4): 419–36.

Irvin, Renee A., and John Stansbury. 2004. "Citizen Participation in Decision Making: Is It Worth the Effort?" *Public Administration Review* 64 (1): 55–65.

King, Cheryl Simrell, Camilla Stivers, and Collaborators. 1998. *Government Is Us: Public Administration in an Anti-Government Era.* Thousand Oaks, CA: Sage.

King, Cheryl Simrell, Kathy M. Feltey, and Bridget O'Neill Susel. 1998. "The Question of Participation: Toward Authentic Participation in Public Decisions." *Public Administration Review* 58 (4): 317–26.

Kweit, Mary G., and Robert W. Kweit. 2004. "Citizen Participation and Citizen Evaluation in Disaster Recovery." *American Review of Public Administration* 34 (4): 354–73.

Lukensmeyer, Carolyn J., and Steven Brigham. 2002. "Taking Democracy to Scale: Creating a Town Hall Meeting for the Twenty-first Century." *National Civic Review* 91 (4): 351–66.

MacNair, R.H., R. Caldwell, and L. Pollane. 1983. "Citizen Participation in Public Bureaucracies: Foul-weather Friends." *Administration and Society* 14: 507–23.

McSwite, O.C. 1997. *Legitimacy in Public Administration: A Discourse Analysis.* Thousand Oaks, CA: Sage.

Roberts, Nancy. 2004. "Public Deliberation in an Age of Direct Citizen Participation." *American Review of Public Administration* 34 (4): 315–53.

Thomas, John C. 1995. *Public Participation in Public Decisions.* San Francisco: Jossey-Bass.

Van Meter, E.C. 1975. "Citizen Participation in the Policy Management Process." *Public Administration Review* 35: 804–12.

Wang, XiaoHu. 2001. "Assessing Public Participation in U.S. Cities." *Public Performance and Management Review* 24 (4): 322–36.

Wang, XiaoHu, and Montgomery Van Wart. 2007. "When Public Participation in Administration Leads to Trust: An Empirical Assessment of Managers' Perceptions." *Public Administration Review* 67 (2): 265–78.

Yang, Kaifeng. 2005. "Public Administrators' Trust in Citizens: A Missing Link in Citizen Involvement Efforts." *Public Administration Review* 65 (3): 273–85.

———. 2006. "Trust and Citizen Involvement Decisions: Trust in Citizens, Trust in Institutions, and Propensity to Trust." *Administration and Society* 38 (5): 573–95.

Yang, Kaifeng, and Kathe Callahan. 2007. "Citizen Involvement Efforts and Bureaucratic Responsiveness: Participatory Values, Stakeholder Pressures and Administrative Practicality." *Public Administration Review* 67 (2): 249–64.

———. 2005. "Assessing Citizen Involvement Efforts by Local Governments." *Public Performance and Management Review* 29 (2): 191–216.

Yang, Kaifeng, and Marc Holzer. 2006. "The Performance-Trust Link: Implications for Performance Measurement." *Public Administration Review* 66 (1): 114–26.

Part II

Democracy and Engagement through Different Lenses

The chapters in Part II examine the possibilities for citizen engagement in public administration through various lenses. As they do so, they address the dilemmas of citizen engagement outlined in Part I and provide diverse ways of considering them. These chapters indicate that we need to step back from the question of whether or not to engage, ask some bigger questions, and even take the questions themselves to task.

Kelly Campbell Rawlings and Tom Catlaw call into question the centrality of situating engagement (a democratic process) in public administration. They argue that lines are blurred between who governs and where as well as between work, home, and life, so that they "see a societal landscape that has changed in ways that pose profound challenges both for public administration theory and practice and serious questions for democracy as we traditionally understand it" (page 32). As such, they suggest that "the scope of the challenge presented to us today is such that a deep reconsideration of public administration in a democracy is needed" (page 33). In their view, it's not enough to respond to the challenges of our current times—to the vacuous and failing practices of democracy—by calling for more engagement and less marketplace or by defending the legitimacy of public administration. This chapter presents the well-formed and lively argument that re-enlivening democracy requires us to live democratically and interrogate our assumptions about what that means.

Richard Box's chapter continues with the interrogation. He situates his argument in the question of whether administrators are neutral implementers of public policy or engaged actors and facilitators in democratic processes. He suggests we do away with the false dichotomy and that administrators are both these things. He examines the concept of citizen self-governance from three perspectives—elite, democratic, and efficiency—and suggests that we can't always fully involve citizens. The second section of his chapter examines citizen involvement in a historical context and shows how difficult it can be to engage citizens in the face of powerful interests, an apathetic public, and the distractions of contemporary life. In the end, he suggests two ways that public professionals can bring citizens' perspectives to the table, even if citizens are not there. As he says, "'Imagining private lives' suggests a way to use knowledge

30

of current conditions that is especially helpful in the absence of public involvement, and 'imagining alternative futures' describes a process for envisioning a future that is not entirely bound by the past" (page 61).

Lisa Zanetti's chapter situates empathy, a value she argues is essential to public service and to improving citizen–government relationships, in the poignant and personal story of her diagnosis and treatment for cancer. Practicing micrology—an explicitly critical and feminist practice of self-reflective interplay between the analytic and the subjective-personal—she draw similarities between illness and disaster recovery and argues that empathy is a value that can stand against American's tendency toward rugged individualism. Because public servants function as mediators between and within all the blurred lines Rawlings and Catlaw outline in their chapter, public administrators are in the unique position to be active sustainers of empathy as a normative value and can build spaces for, as well as model to others, what Zanetti calls "mutual acts of kindness" (page 83).

Mary Timney revives and revises her chapter from the first edition of *Government Is Us* and outlines models of citizen participation and collaboration. She harkens back to the models she presented in the previous edition and revises her perspective given what she's learned about participation and collaboration from observing practice. She provides a scorecard for participation and shows how it relates to an Effective Community Governance Model that includes engaging citizens, measuring results, and getting things done. She also provides suggestions for how to use the scorecard to evaluate citizen participation. Timney's work gives us a way to bridge performance measurement and citizen participation and provides ways to gather empirical data to continue on our quest to learn more about effective collaborative governance.

Jennifer Alexander presents a case study of democratic governance practiced in a nonprofit, in the tradition of the settlement house movement, and shows how it positively affected a county human service agency in crisis. Alexander indicates that the nonprofit literature is rife with the benefits of partnerships from an instrumental perspective. What is ignored is the substantial contribution partnerships can make toward democratic governance and to, in her words, "resolve the challenge of governance failure, defined not in the context of a market model, but as the failure of the public sector to successfully establish relationships of trust and accountability" (page 101). She gives us an alternative way to define accountability: "confidence on the part of citizens that government will act in their best interests, or take action in accordance with shared values" (Ibid.). Her chapter shows how democratic ends and the improvement in citizen–government relationships not only can be attained in organizations outside of government, but may even require an extragovernmental environment, especially with traditionally marginalized populations who believe they haven't seen anything good from the government for a long time, if ever.

3

Democracy as a Way of Life

Rethinking the Places and Practices of Public Administration

Kelly Campbell Rawlings and Thomas Catlaw

> *We may not be able to stop all evil in the world, but I know that how we treat one another, that's entirely up to us.*
> —Barack Obama, Tucson, Arizona (January 12, 2011)

For the last three decades public administration has been grappling with at least two fundamental and intertwined challenges to the foundations of its guiding theories and practices. First, there is widespread recognition that the conventional divisions between the public, private, and nonprofit sectors are blurring. More and more of the work of public policy formulation and service delivery is taking place outside the realm of the government bureau through partnerships, contracts, interagency agreements, and various forms of networked arrangements (Kjaer 2004; Rhodes 1996; Stoker 1998). While, of course, there remain legal and institutional differences among, for example, public and private organizations, an important consequence of this blurring is that the societal division of labor that sectoral distinctions represented is increasingly problematic. The work of traditional politics and administration and the provision of public goods are now clearly happening—and acknowledged to be happening—in the private and nonprofit spheres. In conjunction with this expansion of the realm of politics, greater numbers of citizens, advocacy groups, and other stakeholders are playing vital roles in the daily work of governing. This all makes pinpointing the location of the work of governing and government more difficult. In a telling metaphor, Denhardt and Denhardt (2003) illustrate the two dimensions of this challenge: "The game of public policy formation is no longer played primarily by those in government. You might even say that now the audience is no longer in the stands, but right there on the field, participating in every play" (84).

A second, and related, challenge to public administration theory and practice concerns the growing consciousness that conventional governmental and political action is enabled in profound ways by the patterns of interaction in civil society, home, and work. As one group of scholars put it, "Both the motivation and the capacity to take part in politics have their roots in the fundamental non-political institutions with which individuals are associated during the course of their lives" (Brady, Verba, and Schlozman 1995, 3). In other words, our inclinations to participate and our abilities when we do participate in traditionally defined political life are substantively forged *outside* of the conventional realm of politics. Perhaps the most widely read evidence of this comes from Robert Putnam's (1993) study of governance and civic traditions in Italy. Putnam showed how the relative effectiveness of northern and southern Italian state governments was substantially grounded in the different kind of civic relationships, or social capital, present in each state. In effect, contrary to the idea of civil society as the arena *beyond* government where different interests contest one another and stand in contrast to the "universal" or public interest of government (e.g., "the people"), the civil sphere itself is a significant resource for government; the state is embedded in and enmeshed with civil society, not apart from or above it (Bang and Sørensen 1999).

When we consider these two challenges in light of others—such as the blurring of personal and public space or the meshing of personal and work life facilitated by technology—we see a societal landscape that has changed in ways that pose profound challenges for public administration theory and practice and serious questions for democracy as we traditionally understand it. This traditional way of viewing democracy can be thought of in terms of what Fox and Miller (1995) call the "democratic representative accountability feedback loop." In this scenario, the people express their preferences through the election of representatives, who formulate policy and then pass these policy directives on to public administrators for implementation. The people respond to these implemented policies, and this is fed back to elected officials, who are held accountable through elections for their responsiveness. While this has always been a problematic model of democratic government as matter of practice, today the open and dispersed nature of governance described earlier makes it implausible even as a model.

The question then is how to think and interact "democratically" in this transformed landscape. In many respects, the response of the public administration academic community has been to mount spirited, sophisticated defenses of the public sector; critiques of the pervasiveness of economics and its negative effects on democratic values and public institutions; and to try to fashion new identities, practices, and theories of democratic administration in these dynamic, uncertain conditions. Indeed the first edition of *Government*

Is Us (King, Stivers, and Collaborators 1998) marked a major collective effort toward these ends. Meanwhile, public administration practitioners have been working on the ground to reconcile in innovative ways the ever-growing demands to be increasingly responsive to and inclusive of multiple service partners and citizen groups while maintaining high levels of accountability, efficiency, effectiveness, and transparency in the face of mounting fiscal pressures and political polarization.

In our view, the scope of the challenge presented to us today is such that a deep reconsideration of public administration in a democracy is needed. Defenses of the dignity of public service and the legitimacy of government and charges to hold back the logic of the marketplace or to actively engage the citizenry—all important efforts—are not enough. Rather, on this new landscape the governing of our society needs reconsideration from the ground up; from the very basic practices of everyday life and the manifold interactions and relationships that reside there. In this chapter, we propose a modest contribution to this end. We do not argue for or against a certain normative view, defense, or theory of government per se, but rather seek to describe certain possibilities of *living democratically*. We suggest that democratic self-governing entails a primary focus on the concrete ways in which people talk and live together rather than an ascription of values, functions, and roles to specific institutions, spheres, or sectors of society—all of which have been rendered quite problematic.

This is an idea with a long, rich history (Green 1999), and we take a phrase from the American pragmatist philosopher John Dewey ([1939] 1988) as our starting point. Dewey suggested that beyond our traditional political institutions, mechanisms, and professional duties, "democracy is a *personal* way of individual life" (226). It is a way of life "controlled by personal faith in day by day working together with others" (228). More recently, but to a similar point, John Dryzek (2007) writes that reinvigorating democratic practice today entails "not the spread of liberal democracy to more corners of the world. . . . Instead, it means deepening of the democratic qualities of any situation, structure, or process" (270). Robert Denhardt (1981) has called for the "democratization of social relationships of all types" (634), and other scholars in public administration have also begun to explore this broader view of democratic practice (Al-Yayha et al. 2008; Bryer et al. 2009).

In this chapter, we begin by exploring generally what "democracy as a way of life" means and what its implications are. We then provide some suggestive evidence from social research about why the nonsegmented and integrated view of political life (living-democratically) makes sense by showing how the patterns of interaction in one aspect of our lives really do have an impact on how we think and interact in other aspects. These interconnections are complex, and drawing straightforward causal relations and correlations is not easy—and may not even be possible. Still, existing empirical research helps to make a plausible case for why democratic self-government might usefully be thought of in a more expansive manner, namely as a *way of life.*

Finally, we wish to say that, while we will consider some implications for public administration practice in the conclusion, this chapter is less written for professional public administrators (though we hope they will find it interesting) than for anyone who seeks a reconsideration and rearrangement in the ways in which we live together. As we hope will become clear, this is consistent with the idea of democracy as a way of life and the implication that in the contemporary world, as one of us (Catlaw 2007) has written, "We are all practitioners now" (196). As we will not advance a normative theory of government, we also will not ask the reader to adopt our values or enjoin you to go someplace and "participate." We do not intend a blueprint or cookbook that will tell anyone how to raise their child or run their organization. We rather offer this chapter as another way to think about democratic self-governing, our world and relationships with each other, and to consider the kind of action that might be possible and that makes sense for the reader wherever she or he sits.

Not Just a Form of Government, but Democracy as a Way of Life

The institutions of the modern democratic government, such as elections and voting or constitutions and the rule of law, are the most familiar and most venerable expressions of "democracy" for most of us.[1] In conjunction with these institutions, we invoke certain values like fairness, equality, justice, participation, and freedom in relationship to democracy. Indeed, as Held (2006) explains, it is democracy that connects and binds these values because "the idea of democracy . . . does not just represent one value among many, such as liberty, equality or justice, but it is the value that can link and mediate among competing prescriptive concerns . . . it suggests a way of relating values to each other and of leaving the resolution of value conflicts open to participants in a public process, subject only to certain provisions protecting the shape and form of the process itself" (261).

The idea of democracy as a *way of life,* however, aims at something broader or even more fundamental than these familiar institutions and values. From this vantage, it is *everyday democratic living* that actually gives meaning and content to our democratic values and undergirds the vibrancy of democratic institutions. Dewey's ([1939] 1988) 1939 speech, "Creative Democracy—The Task before Us," captured this expanded sense of democracy. Dewey said that thinking about democracy as a way of life goes beyond traditional conceptualizations and understandings of democracy as a system or form of government and instead considers democracy as "primarily a mode of associated living, of cojoint communicated experience" (Lacey 2008, 123). To think of democracy as a way of life is to infuse democratic practices or logics into all aspects of our everyday lives and to think beyond formal rules of engagement, specified political spheres or sectors, and traditional forms of political participation, like voting. Instead, "democracy" becomes a tangible way to experience, live, and act with others in our day-to-day lives.

Implicit in the idea of democracy as a way of life is the assumption that our lives are intertwined in at least two important ways. First, a person is not a solitary figure going about his or her day in isolation from others. As individuals, we are embedded in dynamic social networks. In discussing Sheldon Wolin's views on democracy, Lacey (2008) explains his view that "'A political being' is not 'an abstract, disconnected bearer of rights, privileges, and immunities' but rather, a 'person whose existence is located in a particular place and draws its sustenance from circumscribed relationships: family, friends, church, neighborhood, workplace, community, town, city.' The identity of a political being is contextual, inseparable from experiences he shares with others in his community" (173–74). Second, our actions and experiences in one arena affect who we are and what we are capable of doing in another. While we will explore this idea in great detail, consider here, for example, how we take our work home with us in much more than a literal sense, or how we expect that the experiences children have in school will have important consequences beyond the classroom. In short, we acquire habits, abilities, and dispositions in certain areas of life that we take with us to other various parts of our lives and that influence what we can do there.

Together, these ideas suggest that what we are able to do, individually and collectively, is a product of the quality of the relationships we have and the ways in which the different areas of our lives are organized. Agency, or our ability to act in the world, is a social product. Lichterman (2009) calls the ability to "do things together" *social capacity,* "the defining feature of [which] is the ability to talk and act reflectively, to coordinate and engage in problem solving that may well involve state or market actors as well as civic ones and include a variety of socially diverse groups and people" (847). Cultivation of this social capacity and democracy as a way of life, then, calls us to examine and be accountable for how our patterns of interaction between and among these various areas and relationships influence each other.

Furthermore, while life is characterized by different interacting relationships, spheres, and arenas, we believe that each of these spaces is meaningfully *political.* As Lacey (2008) puts it, "To become a way of life for all citizens,

36   KELLY CAMPBELL RAWLINGS AND THOMAS CATLAW

democracy has to reach every nook and cranny of our culture, including the family, the school, industry, and religion. Still more, it has to penetrate our souls" (102). With this in mind, it becomes apparent that the very idea of political "participation" changes according to the democracy-as-a-way-of-life perspective. Because democracy is not something happening outside of ourselves or a place or poll we have to go to, no unique or delineated space for democratic interaction need be invented or traveled to. We are always participating in each others' lives (Catlaw and Jordan 2009), and, as such, we can find democratic moments or opportunities within our everyday lives—in our interactions, conversations, attitudes, and actions.

As we suggested in the introduction to this chapter, these everyday democratic interactions matter because they create the conditions necessary to foster or inhibit the growth of a more democratic society in general. In fact, formal institutional democracy *depends* on the everyday actions and interactions of individuals and groups. As Dewey ([1939] 1988) advocated, "unless democratic habits of thought and action are part of the fiber of the people, political democracy is insecure. It cannot stand in isolation. It must be buttressed by the presence of democratic methods in all social relationships" (225). A robust and vibrant democracy does not rely solely on rules of law, periodic voting, and institutionalized structures for governing as is typically thought. It depends as much, if not more so, on what is happening in homes, neighborhoods, schools, places of worship, and workplaces, and the kind of individual agency and social capacity being developed there.

In sum, democracy as a way of life aims to create and sustain a more intentional way of living democratically. It emphasizes the interrelated nature of our individual experiences and lives and how our ability to act individually and together depends on those relationships. Democracy in this sense involves the development of a cooperative spirit among members of a community (however defined) in determining how to go about the everyday work of shared living.

What Is Needed for Democracy as a Way of Life?

But what *are* these democratic practices, dispositions, and interactions that can be supported, reinforced, negated, or absent in our everyday experiences and interactions? In this section, we explore the kinds of attitudes, skills, and capacities that are needed in order to practice democracy as a way of life and we consider some of the ways in which these things are learned, nurtured, and sustained. A wealth of research exists that examines the kinds of skills, capacities, and knowledge needed to participate in political or public life (e.g., Verba, Lehman Schlozman, and Brady 1995; Balch 1974; Battistoni

1997; King et al. 1998; Carpini 2000). The fields of political science, public administration, social psychology, nonprofit studies, and sociology (to name a few) have all approached this notion of what we will call "democratic capacity" in a several ways.

Some researchers (Buchy and Race 2001; Hurtado et al. 2002; Couto 1998; Cooke 2000) have looked at the intrapersonal skills necessary for public and democratic participation. They identify empathy, empowerment, critical awareness, personal development, and maturity as key ingredients. Others examine what can be categorized as political capacity, which includes a concern for equality, fairness, justice, and inclusion as well as a personal sense of efficacy and knowledge of current affairs and the ways in which a political system works (Finkel 1985; Jeffres, Atkin, and Neuendorf 2002; Perry and Katula 2001; Rimmerman 1997). Kirlin (2003) highlights four broad categories of "civic skills" commonly discussed and studied in the literature: organization skills, communication skills, collective decision-making skills, and critical thinking skills. Theoretically, it is assumed that in order to actively participate in public life and civic affairs, a person needs to be able to organize, communicate, engage in collective decision making, and think critically and reflectively. But, as suggested earlier, it is not only the traditional political realm that benefits when individuals possess and make use of these democratic capacities. Moreover, the traditional political or public sphere is not the only location within which these things can be learned, developed, and practiced.

Some caution regarding "off the shelf" cookbook (see Farmer 2005, 83) inventories of skills, values, and capacities is in order, however. The situational, interactional nature of democracy as a way of life necessarily implies a flexibility regarding what words like "justice" and "fairness" or "knowledge of the political system" actually *mean* in a given context. The content of values cannot simply be taken for granted but, as David Farmer (2005) suggests regarding justice, are better viewed as elements in an ongoing process of *seeking* wisdom and understanding. Similarly, "relevant" political knowledge cannot be determined in the abstract (Catlaw 2006c). For example, if we are concerned about how to deal with potentially community-threatening cracks in a dam (see Schmidt 1993), knowledge of the political system may not provide the information most immediately useful. However openness to the experientially gained practical knowledge of grouters would be essential. A certain kind of knowledge, such as technical expertise, also might be used to exclude certain kinds of people from the outset. Indeed a narrowly defined "competency" regarding "complex" administration is precisely one of the most conspicuous ways in which citizens are routinely excluded from governmental processes and is more likely to shut down the kind of open, critical engagement that seems necessary for democratic practice (McSwite 2005). "Maturity" also may be a way to exclude children, youth, or people with mental illness from involvement in matters that affect them quite intimately and on which they are very likely to have practical expertise. So, while inventories of values and aptitudes may be useful starting points for thinking about these practices, they do not substitute for and cannot preempt the ongoing, creative seeking upon which democratic capacity depends.

Making Democracy a Way of Life: Habits, Intersections, and Interconnections

Citizens of a polity are created, not born. We are shaped and influenced in subtle and not so subtle ways by the physical places, institutional interactions, and personal relationships that we encounter throughout our lives. Given this, living democratically is not something we just inherently know how to do. Instead, democratic skills and habits are developed through repetition and practice in the worlds we encounter. But what determines whether a particular skill becomes a habit or reflex? Quite simply: Creating democratic habits and capacities requires *practice*. As Lacey (2008) writes, "The degree to which we perform our action with uninterrupted frequency determines how deeply the tendency becomes ingrained in us. Each one of us embodies these engrained habits, and they in turn define who we are. If we do not cultivate our own habits willfully and instead let them grow willy-nilly or leave them to wilt and die, we fail to live up to our capacity as human beings" (75).

The efficacy of practice and habit, however, also depends on the availability of opportunities to explore, enhance, and test them. Anyone who has ever tried to learn a foreign language has personal knowledge of this. Book and classroom learning are necessary but insufficient if one wants to develop mastery of the language. Practicing in the local, living language is essential. And even once some degree of mastery has been attained, it can fade quickly if not used regularly. Likewise, professional athletes' skills dull after very short breaks from activity; hence the importance of training camps after long, recuperative breaks. Another familiar experience may help to illustrate this matter in a different way. Many of us have gone off to school, church, or workplace retreats at some pleasant mountain, resort, or off-site location. We engage in dialogue and personal exploration, build new relationships, and emerge energized and optimistic about changing the world. It is often dismaying that the world we left behind has not changed with us, and we usually fall back into old habits because the old setting doesn't support or reinforce the new possibilities.

Democracy as a way of life brings this dilemma into sharp relief. Like other habits, democratic habits, skills, and dispositions can be discovered, developed, and encouraged in our homes, schools, churches, workplaces, and so forth. Where there is resonance across various settings, democracy tends to beget more democracy; we learn to participate by participating. But nondemocratic practices similarly tend to replicate and reinforce themselves. For example, when we participate in a team project at work, we can learn about cooperation and practice collective decision making. Conversely, our experiences at work may allow little opportunity to create or to have input into key decisions if we are competing for the scarce positions and resources that affect our livelihoods. When a nonprofit organization engages stakeholders in strategic planning sessions, participants can practice or experience inclusion and learn how to communicate and work with a diversity of perspectives and opinions; alternatively the "leadership team" might make all the decisions and pass on instruction to staff.

In light of the circular or recursive nature of the development of practice and habit, it is important that we pay attention to the nature of relationships and experiences in order to determine what these spaces are currently teaching us and what they could be doing to foster a democratic way of life. This is an idea shared by Dewey who believed "we can only hope to bring abut a 'more equitable and enlightened social order' if a democratic education reaches 'all agencies and influences that shape disposition,' and if 'every place in which men habitually meet—shop, club, factory, saloon, church, political caucus— is perforce a school house, even though not so labeled" (quoted in Lacey 2008, 121). In *Voice and Equality: Civic Voluntarism in American Politics* (1995), which is one of the more extensive studies on civic participation and volunteerism, Verba, Schlozman, and Brady make a similar argument that the "acquisition of [civic] skills depends upon the level of skill opportunity provided by the domain; the extent to which involvement in the domain is socially structured; and the extent to which opportunities for skill development are socially structured among those affiliated" (320).

What follows next is our attempt to identify examples of these democratic practices and an exploration of the effects these practices have on the various relationships and realms in which we take part. Our goal is to connect some of the dots in a way that makes the larger picture of democracy as a way of life more clear and compelling.

The Tangle of Everyday Practices

How do the patterns of relationship and interaction in one domain of life influence the pattern of interaction in other parts of our lives? What are the political "spillover" effects of these interactions? We look at this tangle of everyday practice through the lenses of three important societal modern

40 KELLY CAMPBELL RAWLINGS AND THOMAS CATLAW

institutional spaces—the family, the school, and the workplace. In doing so, we draw contrasts between various kinds of practices and interactions and their broader political effects. We acknowledge at the outset that we cannot provide coverage of all the possible combinations and permutations of interactions and relationships and that the empirical support for many of the points we present is hardly overwhelming. We hope, however, that this discussion provides enough evidence to render the idea of democracy as a way of life as plausible and worthy of further exploration and discussion.

The Family

Our most intimate experience with participation and shared living originates within our families. For this reason, the nature of these relationships and experiences are important to the larger democratic polity. According to Dewey, families and neighborhoods are "the means by which dispositions are stably formed and ideas acquired which laid hold on the roots of character" (Lacey 2008, 105). Through everyday interactions, individuals within families are developing (or suppressing) their abilities to act, to contribute to the general well-being and stability of the family unit, to communicate, to collaborate and compromise, to make decisions, to identify and develop common goals, and to consider and evaluate various outcomes. Herd and Meyer (2002) make the compelling argument that these kinds of activities have the potential to foster and develop the "social and reciprocal ties between individuals [that] is arguably the most important outcome of civic engagement, particularly for social capitalists" (675).

During Dewey's era, many Progressives attempted to employ his ideas and create democratic households. One of the more well-known cases is the Gilbreth family, the subject of the book *Cheaper by the Dozen* by Frank B. Gilbreth Jr. and Ernestine Gilbreth Carey ([1948] 2002). The Gilbreths instituted a home training regimen to teach their children about group responsibility, consumerism, and efficiency methods. (The Gilbreth parents, Frank and Lillian, were both industrial engineers and were devotees of Frederick Taylor and his "scientific management." Lillian is often considered one of the founders of modern management and was an advisor to five U.S. presidents.) One of their democratic family practices was a "Family Council," which "met after Sunday dinner to decide on family policy, which included 'the opening of the work plan and schedules . . . and the educating of the children to the responsibilities they were supposed to assume, the work they had to do and the records they were required to keep'" (Lancaster 2004).

The practices of the family, though, need not encourage democracy; they can help advance other ways of living. In his critical studies of the family and

DEMOCRACY AS A WAY OF LIFE   41

authority, sociologist Max Horkheimer (1972) contended that the patriarchal structure of the family prepared children for the hierarchical world of the capitalist workplace; it is the "germ cell" of this order (128). He argued that a naturalness of paternal power emerges because of "its twofold foundation in the father's economic position and his physical strength with its legal backing" (107). He continued that because of the changes in the economic order, the family order, too, has changed from being a productive community to a consumer community. In this new setting,

> every bourgeois father may in social life have a very modest social position and have to bend the knee to others, yet at home will be a master and exercise the highly important functions of accustoming his children to discretion and obedience. This is why not only the upper middle classes but many groups of workers and employees yield ever new generations of people who do not question the structure of the economic and social system but accept it as natural and permanent and even allow even their dissatisfaction and rebellion to be turned into effective forces for the prevailing order. (108)

Education in the family is "doubtless the most effective preparation for such surrender of individual volition" (110), which is an essential feature of the efficient capitalist enterprise and also an important precondition for the rise of the totalitarian state. However, Horkheimer believed that at the same time, the family offered a kind of respite from the world of market relations, a place where a person potentially could be a human being rather than a mere function, and this provided the capacity to imagine and dream of another, better life (114).[2] But he was pessimistic that any change could occur in this submissive attitude toward authority until the underlying structure of the family eroded (112).

The relation between the family and workplace is a critical one, but, without discounting the instrumental relationship of the government and economy vis-à-vis the family, it is likely more bidirectional or recursive than what Horkheimer suggests. Parents bring habits and patterns of interaction and affect to the workplace and also take them home to their children (Eby, Maher, and Butts 2010; Ritchie 1997) as they seek to prepare their offspring for society through their own experiences. Anthropological evidence shows that "family relations and expectations [influence] people's choices or actions in changing economic contexts" yet economic changes also condition or necessitate experimentation in family relations (Creed 2000, 333). For example, the post–World War II economic boom facilitated the appearance of the so-called "traditional" family by providing economic and social conditions for "early marriage, early childbearing, consumer debt, and big houses in the suburbs" (335).

Related to this, family forms also may affect the workplace and government as idealized images and metaphors for structuring interactions in those sites. The cognitive scientist George Lakoff (2002) has written that American politics is essentially oriented around two competing narrative responses to the metaphor of the nation as family. He shows how conservatives advance a "strict father" model whereas liberals promote a "nurturing parent" one. The postwar image of the nuclear family described here also helped to mobilize economic and social policies that would sustain the American Dream. Family forms have also been transposed to the workplace as models for paternalistic supervisor-staff relationships or care and cooperation (Bauman 2000; Creed 2000; Stivers 2000). As the economic crisis of the twenty-first century unfolds, it will be interesting to see whether new family forms emerge and if there are changes in peoples' interactions with authority.

Research in political science has examined the influence of the family on political activity or efficacy later in life. In general, this work suggests that if parents are civically engaged, children are more likely to be as well (see Campbell 2006, chapter 5; Mettler 2002; Kentand Jennings and Niemi 1981; Verba, Schlozman, and Brady 1995), though children from homes of a higher socioeconomic status (SES) are more likely to become civically active than children with lower SES.[3] Patterns of everyday interaction also matter, such as parent-child discussions about politics and community activity (McFarland and Thomas 2006). Two things seem important in this regard. First, information about politics, such as poll location, candidates' positions, and electoral processes (McFarland and Thomas 2006) is transmitted but so too is a form of talk and interaction. For example, research in communication (Kohn 1977) suggests that parents may interact with their children in one of two general ways. The first emphasizes obedience to authority and discipline on the basis of outcomes rather than intentions; the second focuses on the autonomy and self-direction of the child and openness and mental flexibility on the part of the parent. Thus, while the transmission of information or content is relevant, so is the form or way in which the child learns to learn.[4]

But we would do well to remember that children and adolescents are not simplistically imprinted with "family values" (see, for example, Persson, Stattin, and Kerr 2004). Children also help to structure the family through their interactions with media, peers, schools, and other institutions. So, as social dynamics continue apace in the twenty-first century, we should expect new habits and dispositions among young people that will emerge as they adapt and respond to new familial arrangements and the expectations of the varied worlds they encounter to, in the words of Schwartz (1987), "jointly construct [with adults] the moral and social fabric of the common culture" (5).

The School

While the family clearly plays an important role in cultivating and reproducing certain patterns of interaction, the family is not destiny and, with regard to later political activities, there may be a tendency to overestimate the monopoly of early childhood experiences with regard to the formation of specific opinions (Mason 1982, 81–82). Other institutional settings also play roles in developing habits and in activating (or not activating) capacities or dispositions learned elsewhere or in reinforcing certain kinds of relationships. The school is an important one.

There is a wide range of research that has suggested there is a direct correlation between education and levels of public involvement and participation. For example, Emler and Frazer (1999) argue that persons with more education are more likely to be politically active, and Verba, Schlozman, and Brady (1995) revealed that parental education plays a significant role in political activity and socialization; the more education parents have, the more they participate and so the more likely it is that their children will too. Again, these interactions seem to feed on themselves.

In addition to the general effects of education, the structure of the educational experience has long been thought to have broad societal impacts. In a series of lectures given in 1902–3, the French sociologist Emile Durkheim ([1903] 1961) famously described the central role that schools play in teaching morality to young people. He suggested that schools provided a "second childhood" and an education that completed and carried forward—or corrected—the one begun in the family. This was not merely an education that involved the transfer of information or technical knowledge; more importantly, it was a *moral* education that would transfer norms, dispositions, and preferences and prepare children for their future life in the adult order of things. Morality, he said with some hyperbole, is "like so many molds with limiting boundaries, into which we must pour our behavior" (26).

At the root of morality or the "moral temperament," Durkheim contended, was the notion of *discipline* (31), a necessary limiting and bounding spirit (cf. Foucault 1995). This is what he felt the school could provide, even more so than the family (146–48). But Durkheim did not view discipline as inherently limiting or constraining in an absolute sense. Indeed the consequences for society were regularity in social interaction and conscience and, by extension, cohesion. For the individual, the benefit was also an experience of ordered regularity and a sense of social place that defended against what Durkheim called *anomie* or the experience of detachment caused either by the erosion of norms or by excessively rigid norms. In effect, school discipline would help to produce certain kinds of people with specific capacities and moral views of the world. Durkheim said, *"Education creates a new being"* (xiv) in accordance with the needs of society.

For our more modest purposes, the key takeaway from Durkheim's argument is that one particular institutional space, the school, has consequences that reach far beyond its institutional boundaries. The discipline of the school is the way in which society was able to reproduce a morality, a discipline, to its members. It prepared children for the different institutional spaces, such as those in the workplace and civil society, that they would enter (or not enter). However, discipline did not necessarily imply any particular *kind* of discipline. As Durkheim says, "A given teaching method may be totally transformed depending on the way in which it is carried out. . . . [D]iscipline will produce quite different outcomes according to one's conception of its nature and function for life in general and education in particular" (36–7). In effect, different forms of discipline help to produce different kinds of citizens, or different beings.

Some, but certainly not all, Americans during the Progressive era saw the power of the schools to fabricate citizens, particularly *democratic* ones, in a similar light. John Dewey, again, is exemplary in this regard. Dewey [1909] (1959) thought that the school was an institution created to advance the welfare of the community and to train young people for citizenship and active participation in social life. This training, however, involved more than learning about how to vote intelligently or obedience to the law. In light of the many different spheres in which a child will find herself, she needed training or discipline in the arts, history, methods of inquiry, tools for communication, and physical well-being. She needs education for leadership and obedience; the power of self-direction and the direction of others, as well as the ability to be directed (10); and the capacity for intellectual and emotional judgment (52–3). "Discipline is genuinely educative only as it represents a reaction of information into the individual's own powers so that she can bring them under control for social ends" (32). Discipline in a democracy, then, is needed to activate the individual's power for creativity and agency.

Because of the densely interwoven, recursive quality of social life, Dewey thought that "there cannot be two sets of ethical principles, one for life in the school, and the other for life outside the school" (7). He found "every subject, every method of instruction, every incident of school life [to be] pregnant with moral possibility" (58). But rather than a democratic capacity being cultivated, Dewey saw in the schools of the time something like what Horkheimer saw in the family—the development of a spirit of discipline that was at once individualistic and deferential to authority. In absence of social activity that called forth the child's creative possibility, the only real motive for continued study was pleasing the teacher and following rules (23–4).

With Dewey, others worried that the American school system had engaged in "unfortunate borrowing" during the mid-nineteenth century from the Prussian school system, and so was reproducing a kind of class division in schooling—one for aristocrats and one for the common people (Judd 1918). The results for a democratic polity could only be negative.

In discussions on the then-emerging School or Community Centers movement, Mary Follett ([1920] 1998), a contemporary of Dewey's, said that the purpose of education was to "fit children for the life of the community" and very clearly echoed Durkheim's argument. She said, "When we change our ideas of the relation of the individual to society, our whole system of education changes. What we want to teach is interdependence, that efficiency waits on discipline, that discipline is obedience to the whole of which I am a part. Discipline has been a word long connected with school life—when we know how to teach social discipline then we shall know how to 'teach school'" (63). Discipline for a democracy entailed learning how to work with others and, in doing so, discover and contribute one's own point of view and difference. This was training for democratic citizenship that had at its center the cultivation of the ability to "meet the clash of differences . . . which life brings" (365). Such training, she said, could not be left to mere evolution but needed to be deliberate. Group activities, civics courses, and experiences in self-government (such as school councils or young people's civic clubs) ought to pervade a child's in-school and after-school life. She emphasized, "And it must be remembered that the chief value of these clubs is not the information acquired, not even the interest aroused, but the lesson learned from genuine discussion with all the advantages therefrom" (369). For Dewey, a democratic moral education needed to be learned through democratic means; democratic knowledge needed to be created democratically.

It is precisely because most people still believe, as Durkheim, Dewey, and Follett did, that schools *do* transmit more than inert, technical information to children that we find schools and education generally at the center of many of our most contentious political disputes. But while social theory and our political intuitions support these ideas, empirical support for precisely what is transmitted and how it impacts adult life has been surprisingly limited.

One excellent example, though, comes from Daniel McFarland and Reuben Thomas (2006), who examined the ways in which extracurricular activities affect political involvement later in life (e.g., voting, involvement in presidential campaigns, volunteering in community or civic organization). In examining two large, longitudinal data sets, they found compelling evidence that "involvement in politically salient youth voluntary associations has significant, positive returns on adult political participation seven to twelve years later." Specifically they found that National Honor Society, service clubs, student

46   KELLY CAMPBELL RAWLINGS AND THOMAS CATLAW

council, drama clubs, musical groups, and religious groups all had positive effects on involvement later in life (412). (Interestingly, classes in government and civics did not have such effects.[5]) What did youth learn in these activities? More or less what Dewey and Follett thought they would: "public speaking, debate, community service, communal representation, which in turn develop relations, skills, knowledge, identities, and interest in political systems that hold over into adulthood" (418). That is, they develop a social spirit and the individual capacities necessary to act, explore, and advance that spirit. Family life, though, matters because, once again, comparatively advantaged students in terms of SES and the educational attainment of their parents "disproportionately use these pathways" (421).

It cannot be denied, though, that while many have hoped for and explored the democratic potential of school (Apple and Beane 1999; Dobozy 2007; Gutmann [1987] 1999) and McFarland and Thomas's research indicates that this potential sometimes is realized, the reality is often quite different. There is another kind of social reproduction underway, one that remains distinctly *undemocratic* and *unequal*. Today scholars call attention to the significant disparities across class and race and how they express themselves in schoolplace disciplining. Samuel Bowles and Herbert Gintis (1977), for example, describe the ways in which the structure of the school and its formal positions (administrator, teacher, student) prepare students for the division of labor in the modern workplace and to accept relations of subordination. Others call attention to how school interactions replicate existing inequalities in race, gender, and class and related cultural practices and valuations which, again, habituates students to accept these as natural or given when they see them in the adult world of work, civic, and political life. Aaron Kupchik and Torin Monahan (2006) argue that the new spaces of schools—with increased technological surveillance and police presence—are preparing youth for the new world of global capitalism, militarization, and mass imprisonment by normalizing the presence of surveillance, police, and the risk of incarceration in everyday life. Indeed, for millions of poor, disproportionately African American youth the socializing function of the school seems to have been abandoned entirely; for them, schools have become places of confinement, warehouses, or alternative kinds of prisons (Wacquant 2001, 2002).

The Workplace

In the 1960s, concern for understanding the effects of relationships in one area of life on another spread beyond the school and family to include the workplace. Among the more prominent and influential accounts of the period was Carol Pateman's (1970) *Participation and Democratic Theory.*[6] Pateman's contention was that much of what she called "contemporary political theory" had defined the nature of democracy in excessively narrow terms. The participation of all in a democratic polity was deemed unrealistic and mythical; expectations needed to be curbed and participatory impulses quelled (see McSwite 1997). Democracy, these scholars contended, should be seen as a particular "method" for the selection of decision makers. Elections thus equate democracy with political representation, defined as relatively open competition for leadership, by and large among elites. Indeed many political theorists came to see the ideal of equal and open participation (beyond voting) as a *threat* to this democratic method and explored ways in which a vertical, hierarchical relationship among elite leadership and the general public could be sustained.

Pateman rejected the claims of contemporary theory on intertwined normative and empirical grounds. She argued that "the theory of participatory democracy is built around the central assertion that individuals and their institutions cannot be considered in isolation from one another" (42). Democracy, she contended, needed to "take place in other spheres in order that the necessary individual attitudes and psychological qualities can be developed. This development takes place through the process of participation itself" (Ibid.). Participation, then, was not the problem its critics thought it was. As we suggested earlier, people did not need to go someplace and discuss every issue. Rather it was a matter of distributing and developing patterns of relationship that encouraged participation in all social settings. In other words, there was not a *single* political system in which people participated, but an array of varied political *systems.* This was an expanded notion of what counted as political space and political interaction (see Catlaw 2007; Denhardt 1968; Golembiewski 1989; Mason 1982).

Given the amount of time and effort modern humans devote to paid employment, Pateman thought that the workplace was the crucial site for developing a democratic polity (see also Denhardt 1981). She then mobilized the empirical evidence to that point (such as it was) about the educative effects of participation and the possibility of democratizing modern workplaces. She concluded that the theoretical tenets of participatory democracy concerning the politically important psychological and educative effects of participation had real empirical support and that greater involvement in decision making and work processes was perceived as desirable by industrial workers. In a kind of sequel to Pateman's text, Ron Mason (1982) explores the theoretical and empirical association of work and political efficacy in some detail and concludes, similarly, that the empirical research, while limited given the importance of the topic, also supports the connection between workplace participation, the development of personal political efficacy, and participation in other forms of political life outside work (100; see also Greenberg, Grunberg, and Daniel 1996).[7]

More concretely, though, we can think about participation and influence in the workplace and democracy on three levels (Adman 2008)[8]: (1) "job autonomy," which speaks to an individual's control over daily work activity; (2) face-to-face interactions concerning the influence an employee has in collective decision making in her proximate work group or team; and (3) the influence employees have in "enterprise level" decision making, or in setting the overall goals, values, and direction of the organization or agency as a whole. Given an ability to influence the direction and content of their work, employees become more than functionaries carrying out orders from above. They gain a stronger sense of self-worth and confidence in dealing with the world, and a sense of being part of something larger than themselves. They are connected to themselves, their work, and the whole.

Through their experiences at work, people also can develop other important skills and abilities that are useful for public participation and civic engagement. Returning to our earlier discussion on intrapersonal capacities, these types of skills and abilities can be classified into three broad categories: organization skills, such as planning, identifying stakeholders, or running an effective meeting; communication skills, such as public speaking, writing, and active listening; and critical thinking skills, like synthesizing and analyzing information (Kirlin 2003). Through workplace participation, employees can also sharpen their decision-making skills and cultivate their collaborating and consensus-building abilities. Importantly, individuals can foster certain kinds of attitudes through workplace practices and interactions that are congenial (or not) to a democratic polity, such as, most importantly, a sense of justice and fairness. Research on "organizational justice" indicates that employees are quite sensitive to distributive (appropriateness of outcomes), procedural (appropriateness of processes), and interactional justice (appropriateness of treatment from authority) (Cropanzano, Bowen, and Gilliand 2007). Organizations that are managed "justly" are more likely to encourage trust and commitment among employees, and it should come as no surprise that these sentiments spill over into relationships outside the organization.

Democracy and the Workplace: Further Interconnections

We now explore two more relevant dimensions of the political spillover effects of democratic practices in the workplace: (1) how workplace communication patterns influence what happens in the family and (2) how the internal practices of a public organization may influence how public administrators are inclined or disinclined to work with the public.

DEMOCRACY AS A WAY OF LIFE   49

Kohn's (1977) and Kohn and Schooler's (1981) research indicates that when fathers are employed in a workplace that emphasizes conformity and deference to hierarchical authority, both parents are less likely to exhibit "mental flexibility and more likely to express conservative, authoritarian values" (Ritchie 1997, 177). When the structure of the workplace encourages autonomy and individual initiative, both parents are likely to "express greater mental flexibility and to emphasize self-direction and openness" (177). The effects seem to become stronger and mutually reinforce one another over time. The underlying rationale for this, Kohn suggests, is that parents understandably seek to prepare their children for the world that they will encounter. Subsequent work by Kohn and Schooler (1981) and others indicated that the education level (e.g., some college) and the complexity and autonomy associated with housework could also cultivate tendencies for conformity or conversation in mothers who did not work outside the home.

Occupational complexity, autonomy, and educational attainment, in general, seem to encourage the development of an open conversational orientation in parent-child communication (Ritchie 1997). Gender and work relations have changed since some of this research was conducted, however the findings nevertheless support the intuitive notion that parents take more than their work home with them; they also take with them the workplace patterns of communication, affect, and interaction (see also Eby et al. 2010; Lambert 1990; Staines 1980). If openness to dialogue and criticism of authority are important practices for developing democratic capacity, this has relevance for how we organize our workplaces.

Finally, Alkadry (2003) examined whether administrators listen to citizens. Specifically, he sought to explore whether the theoretical critiques of the negative effects of technical rationality and bureaucracy (e.g., alienation; domination; lack of autonomy; one-dimensional, closed thinking) imposed structural constraints on the ability of administrators to act, especially with regard to citizen feedback (188). His findings confirmed "existing theories about the effect of organizational structure on individual behavior" (203).

However Alkadry noted that the removal of bureaucratic constraints would not alone enhance the responsiveness of public administrators since individual administrators also have *personal* constraints to responsiveness rooted in their perceptions of citizens and faith in their own professional expertise. Many other theorists have begun examining this notion of what individual administrators are bringing to the table and the ways in which these attitudes, skills, and knowledge gained through external experiences are influencing and affecting the relationships between administrators and citizens (Yang and Callahan 2005; Kumar, Kant, and Amburgey 2007; Brewer 2003; Bryer 2007; Yang 2005, 2006). Nevertheless, the workplace structures

50 KELLY CAMPBELL RAWLINGS AND THOMAS CATLAW

of some contemporary bureaucracies do indeed seem to have some influence not only on the patterns of communication within the public agency but also on how individual administrators interact with citizens. Closed-off organizations may encourage administrators to have closed-off attitudes toward the publics they serve.

Living Democratically: What Have We Learned?

We conclude this chapter by taking inventory of what we have learned about democracy as a way of life and, more particularly, what the *democracy* in the phrase "living democratically" signifies.

First, while the idea of democracy as a way of life seems simple, once we scratch the surface of the phrase, the reality beneath is quite complex. It is difficult to draw any simple causal relationship between the practices of one institutional setting and democratic practices later in life in the abstract. And it is hard to know how the unique mix of relationships in the familial, educational, and occupational settings (to name only three possible settings) will interact with the experiences and history of any concrete individual. Everyday life is a complex tangle of practices, interactions, and experiences.

Still, we know that the activities in the family, school, and workplace *do* influence the ways in which we interact with one another elsewhere, even if the interactions are complex and difficult to disentangle. More precisely, we find that the development of capacities for future interactions in public, civic, and governmental life are produced in varied and sometimes surprising places and ways. There is little doubt about this and, as such, it does not make sense to limit our notion of politics to a narrow band of life. We also cannot ignore the fact that the positive and negative effects of these democratic interactions and practices and capacity building are unequally distributed. Because of the densely intermeshed nature of social life, these effects also have profound consequences for a democratic polity and our collective well-being. Indeed, the best evidence concerning the spillover effect of democratic practices illustrates the ways in which these benefits accrue to those already disposed to enjoy and make use of them.

We think that this complexity is itself a compelling reason to consider democracy as a way of life and to see the activities of the political in an expansive way. Since we cannot know for certain whether specific settings will help to cultivate democratic habits or whether different settings will put them to work and deepen them, it seems reasonable to seek the development of democratic habits wherever and whenever possible. So we cannot simply rely, for instance, on a public service motivation cultivated in childhood in order to sustain interest in public service. That disposition needs to be nurtured and deepened as people move through the various places and stages of their lives. We should not simply assume that school or university training will prepare students for a life of public service by either overcoming familial habituation or substituting for the presence of democratic practices at work. We cannot saddle families in whatever form they assume with cultivating democratic habits in their children absent enabling, supportive conditions in the workplace, schools, and marketplace. The reality is complex and there is not a neat division of labor that allows us to assign responsibility for democracy to one area of life or another. And though life is complex and fragmented, democracy as a way of life means that we have to take actual human beings as a whole (Farmer 2005) and to act accordingly.

Second, what have we learned about how "democratic" modifies "way of life"? We would say that democracy as we have explored it here refers to a particular qualitative *process* or way of talking and interacting with others. This process emphasizes openness to the other; flexible habits of mind; a concern for individual creativity, autonomy, and personal efficacy; involvement in the tasks close at hand in our lives, which, in turn, seems to facilitate the development of a sense of self in relation to others; and close attention to the concrete empirical situation. It is concerned, to borrow Orion White's nice wording, with the particular *texture* of contextual interaction or contact and a kind of mutual learning through activity and interaction that such contact provides (1990).

Democracy as a way of life is *not* about the abolition of (or total liberation from) authority or power; nor is it a roadmap to Flatland. For example, democracy as a way of life does not appear to demand restructuring families with children, classrooms, or workplaces, though democratic process may lead to such change in specific, concrete cases. Rather it concerns more the particular manner in which authority or power is exercised. Democracy as a way of life does not appear to be necessarily antibureaucratic or pro any other organizational form. Rather, as a *form of life* rather than a kind of organization, it cuts across these divisions and exists as a relational possibility in concrete settings—though much in our contemporary world frustrates its practice.

How, then, might public administrators go about incorporating some of the practices we have explored here? Rather than giving a set of directions, we offer instead several questions that administrators might relate to their work situation. While these are simple, we hope they might serve as a springboard for others: Where in the work process is it possible to use consensus-based decision making?[9] If broad organizational goals are set from above, is it possible to open opportunities for collaboration at the department or group/team level? Where can job autonomy be encouraged or expanded? Are there opportunities for employees to practice and develop organizational, communication,

52 KELLY CAMPBELL RAWLINGS AND THOMAS CATLAW

and critical thinking skills? If distributional justice issues (e.g., compensation and benefits) are beyond the control of the manager, are procedural and interactional matters being attended to? Answering these questions (and others) might go some way toward practicing democracy as a way of life.

Finally we offer a word of caution: "Democracy" today has been elevated to a most exalted, almost untouchable status. It is nearly symptomatic of some political or personal pathology not to be a democrat or to suggest that individuals and humanity may not be intrinsically animated by a hunger for "democracy" (Badiou 2002). It was so in the Progressive era, too (Waldo 1948), which saw Dewey (1927) proclaim that the cure for democracy was more democracy. We do not wish for the kind of life explored here to itself become a club that would beat out of us the very possibility for this type of life. For these reasons, we have sought to detach "democracy" from both its normative ideal and more narrow presentation as a form of government in order to focus on its interactional practice in the daily life that we share with one another.

Notes

The impetus for this chapter has its origins in ongoing conversations with colleagues and friends over many years. We wish to thank, in particular, the participants in the TOC and Participation discussion groups, Khalid Al-Yayha, Michael Coyle, Chao Guo, Qian Hu, and Heather Stickeler; as well members of the Minnowbrook III PA Theory group, Tom Bryer, Angela Eikenberry, Kyle Farmbry, Catherine Horiuchi, Matthew Mingus, Tony Molina, and Margaret Stout. Appreciation is extended to the vigorous participants in the "Democracy as Way of Life" Open Spaces group at the 2009 Public Administration Theory Network conference and to Cheryl King for her persistence and commitment to this project.

1. For a more detailed discussion of the various models of democracy and democratic ideals and aims, see Held 2006.

2. In some respects, Horkheimer's views were confirmed later in psychology research on "compensation theory," which found that employees may invest more time and effort in their family to compensate for dissatisfaction at work (Eby et al. 2010). See also Lambert (1990) for an overview of compensation and spillover in work-family relations.

3. Interest in early childhood and familial experiences is found in public administration research on public service motivation (PSM) (Brewer 2009; Perry 1997, 2000; Perry and Wise, 1990). PSM emerged as a theoretical construct to explore whether there are differences among employees in public, private, and nonprofit organization in terms of the kinds of work they seek and why they do so. In his model of PSM, Perry (2000) takes account of family life in the category of "sociohistorical context."

4. Of course, family structure has changed during the last eighty years or so, especially for less economically and educationally advantaged women who are single parents (McLanahan and Percheski 2008), along with the structure of the capitalist political economy and gender and authority relations in general (Castells 2000; Catlaw

2006a,b; Mitscherlich [1963] 1969). So too have youth attitudes toward authority during this period. Schwartz's (1987) work on youth subcultures since the 1970s, for example, suggests that young people's attitude toward rebellion and authority has shifted markedly. Rebellion was no longer oriented toward rejection of authority or disobeying the law but rather disengagement with conventional definitions of success and responsibility.

5. There is evidence to suggest, however, that education regarding the working of government processes can positively influence citizens' perceptions of government. See Hibbing and Theiss-Morse (2002).

6. Pateman was not alone in her position; nor was interest in workplace democracy new in the 1960s. She drew on the work of G.D.H. Cole, J.S. Mill, and nineteenth-century thinkers, and many then-contemporary organizational theorists, such as Argyris, made similar claims.

7. A more recent empirical investigation is Jian and Jeffres (2008), which looked at both formal aspects of workplace relationships (e.g., job autonomy and involvement in decision making) and informal influences of the workplace community on political activity outside work. Their data suggested that job autonomy and decision involvement is associated with a high sense of personal political effectiveness and, in turn, higher levels of participation in voting, community affairs, and campaign activities. The relationship between decision involvement and voting, though, was found to be direct (i.e., without the mediating effects of internal or personal political efficacy). In explaining this they speculated that "participation in decision making at work cultivates a pattern or habit of involvement in collective events" and sense of duty that "transcends the boundaries between work and politics" (46).

8. The remainder of this section appeared originally in Catlaw and Rawlings (2010, in press).

9. The paragraph appeared originally in Catlaw and Rawlings (2010).

References

Adman, Per. 2008. "Does Workplace Experience Enhance Political Participation? A Critical Test of a Venerable Hypothesis." *Political Behavior* 30 (1):115–38.

Al-Yayha, Khalid, Kelly C. Rawlings, Thomas J. Catlaw, Chao Guo, and Qian Hu. 2008. "Participation: Revolution Recovered." In Panel Presentation at the Annual Conference of the American Society for Public Administration. Dallas, TX.

Alkadry, Mohamad. 2003. "Deliberative Discourse between Citizens and Administrators: If Citizens Talk, Will Administrators Listen?" *Administration & Society* 35 (2): 184–209.

Apple, Michael W., and James A. Beane. 1999. *Democratic Schools: Lessons from the Chalk Face.* Buckingham, UK: Open University Press.

Badiou, Alain. 2002. "Highly Speculative Reasoning on the Concept of Democracy." *The Symptom* 2.

Balch, George I. 1974. "Multiple Indicators in Survey Research: The Concept 'Sense of Political Efficacy.'" *Political Methodology* 1 (Spring): 1–43.

Bang, Henrik P., and Eva Sørensen. 1999. "The Everyday Maker: A New Challenge to Democratic Governance." *Administrative Theory and Praxis* 31 (3): 325–41.

Battistoni, Richard M. 1997. "Service Learning and Democratic Citizenship." *Theory Into Practice* 36 (3): 150.

54   KELLY CAMPBELL RAWLINGS AND THOMAS CATLAW

Bauman, Zygmunt. 2000. *Community: Seeking Safety in an Insecure World.* London: Polity Press.

Bowles, Samuel, and Herbert Gintis. 1977. *Schooling in Capitalist America: Educational Reform and the Contradictions of Economic Life.* New York: Basic Books.

Brady, H.E., Sidney Verba, and K.L. Schlozman. 1995. "Beyond SES: A Resource Model of Political Participation." *American Political Science Review* 89 (2): 271–97.

Brewer, Gene A. 2003. "Building Social Capital: Civic Attitudes and Behavior of Public Servants." *Journal of Public Administration Research and Theory* 13 (1): 5–26.

———. 2009. "Public Service Motivation: Theory, Evidence, and Prospects for Research." Paper presented at Annual Meeting of the American Political Science Association, August 29–September 1, Boston, MA.

Bryer, Thomas A. 2007. "Toward a Relevant Agenda for a Responsive Public Administration." *Journal of Public Administration Research and Theory* 17 (3): 479–500.

Bryer, Thomas, Thomas J. Catlaw, Angela M. Eikenberry, Kyle Farmbry, Catherine Horiuchi, Matthew Mingus, Anthony Molina, and Margaret R. Stout. 2009. "Administrating the Commons: Imagining Public Administration in a Sectorless Society." Unpublished manuscript.

Buchy, Marlene, and Digby Race. 2001. "The Twists and Turns of Community Participation in Natural Resource Management in Australia: What Is Missing?" *Journal of Environmental Planning and Management* 44 (3): 293–308.

Campbell, David E. 2006. *Why We Vote: How Schools and Communities Shape Our Civic Life.* Princeton: Princeton University Press.

Carpini, Michael X. Delli. 2000. "Gen.com: Youth, Civic Engagement, and the New Information Environment." *Political Communication* 17 (4): 341–49.

Castells, Manuel. 2000. *The Rise of Network Society.* 2d ed. London: Blackwell.

Catlaw, Thomas J. 2006a. "Authority, Representation and the Contradictions of Post-traditional Governing." *American Review of Public Administration* 36 (3): 261–87.

———. 2006b. "Discourse, Decision and the Doublet: An Essay on the Crisis of Modern Authority." In *The Handbook of Decision Making,* ed. G. Morcol. London: Taylor & Francis.

———. 2006c. "Performance Anxieties: Shifting Public Administration from the Relevant to the Real." *Administrative Theory and Praxis* 28 (1): 89–120.

———. 2007. *Fabricating the People: Politics and Administration in the Biopolitical State.* Tuscaloosa, AL: University of Alabama Press.

Catlaw, Thomas J., and Greg M. Jordan. 2009. "Public Administration and the 'Lives of Others': Toward an Ethics of Collaboration." *Administration & Society* 41 (3): 290–312.

Catlaw, Thomas J., and Kelly C. Rawlings. 2010. "Promoting Participation from the Inside-Out: Workplace Democracy and Public Engagement." In *Promoting Citizen Engagement and Community Building,* ed. J.V. Denhardt and J.H. Svara. Phoenix, AZ: Alliance for Innovation.

Cooke, Maeve. 2000. "Five Arguments for Deliberative Democracy." *Political Studies* 48 (5): 947.

Couto, Richard A. 1998. "Community Coalitions and Grassroots Policies of Empowerment." *Administration & Society* 30 (5): 569–94.

Creed, Gerald W. 2000. "'Family Values' and Domestic Economies." *Annual Review of Anthropology* 29: 329–59.

Cropanzano, Russell, David E. Bowen, and Stephen W. Gilliand. 2007. "The Management of Organizational Justice." *Academy of Management Perspectives* 21 (4): 34–48.

Denhardt, Janet V., and Robert B. Denhardt. 2003. *The New Public Service: Serving, not Steering.* Armonk, NY: M.E. Sharpe.

Denhardt, Robert B. 1968. "Organizational Citizenship and Personal Freedom." *Public Administration Review* 28 (1): 47–54.

———. 1981. *In the Shadow of Organization.* Lawrence: The Regents Press of Kansas.

Dewey, John. (1909) 1959. *Moral Principles in Education.* New York: Philosophical Library.

———. 1927. *The Public and Its Problems.* New York: Holt.

———. (1939) 1988. "Creative Democracy: The Task before Us." In *John Dewey: The Later Works, 1925–1953,* ed. R.W. Sleep. Carbondale, IL: Southern Illinois Press.

Dobozy, Eva. 2007. "Effective Learning of Civic Skills: Democratic Schools Succeed in Nurturing Capacities of Students." *Education Studies* 33 (2): 115–28.

Dryzek, John S. 2007. "Networks and Democractic Ideals." In *Theories of Democratic Network Governance,* ed. E. Sorensen and J. Torfing, 262–73. London: Palgrave Macmillan.

Durkheim, Emile. (1903) 1961. *Moral Education: A Study in the Theory and Application of the Sociology of Education,* trans. H. Schnurer and E.K. Wilson. Glenco, IL: Free Press.

Eby, Lillian T., Charleen P. Maher, and Marcus M. Butts. 2010. "The Intersection of Work and Family Life: The Role of Affect." *Annual Review of Psychology* 61: 9.1–9.24.

Emler, Nicholas, and Elizabeth Frazer. 1999. "Politics: The Education Effect." *Oxford Review of Education* 25 (1/2): 251–73.

Farmer, David John. 2005. *To Kill the King: Post-Traditional Governance and Bureaucracy.* Armonk, NY: M.E. Sharpe.

Finkel, Steven E. 1985. "Reciprocal Effects of Participation and Political Efficacy: A Panel Analysis." *American Journal of Political Science* 29 (4): 441–64.

Follett, Mary Parker. (1920) 1998. "The Training for a New Democracy." In *The New State: Group Organization, the Solution of Popular Government.* University Park: Pennsylvania State University Press.

Foucault, Michel. 1995. *Discipline and Punish: The Birth of the Prison,* trans. A. Sheridan. 2d ed. New York: Vintage Books.

Fox, Charles J., and Hugh T. Miller. 1995. *Postmodern Public Administration: Toward Discourse.* Thousand Oaks, CA: Sage.

Gilbreth Jr., Frank B., and Elizabeth Gilbreth Carey. (1948) 2002. *Cheaper by the Dozen.* New York: Perennial Classics.

Golembiewski, Robert T. 1989. "Toward Positive and Practical Public Management: Organizational Research Supporting a Fourth Critical Citizenship." *Administration & Society* 21 (2): 200–27.

Green, Judith. 1999. *Deep Democracy: Community, Diversity, and Transformation.* Lanham, MD: Rowman & Littlefield.

Greenberg, Edward S., Leon Grunberg, and Kelley Daniel. 1996. "Industrial Work and

56   KELLY CAMPBELL RAWLINGS AND THOMAS CATLAW

Political Participation: Beyond 'Simple Spillover.'" *Political Research Quarterly* 49 (2): 305–30.

Gutmann, Amy. (1987) 1999. *Democratic Education*. Princeton, NJ: Princeton University Press.

Held, David. 2006. *Models of Democracy*. 3d ed. Cambridge, UK: Polity Press.

Herd, Pamela M., and Madonna H. Meyer. 2002. "Care Work: Invisible Civic Engagement." *Gender & Society* 16 (5): 665–88.

Hibbing, John R., and Elizabeth Theiss-Morse. 2002. *Stealth Democracy: Americans' Beliefs about How Government Should Work*. Cambridge, UK: Cambridge University Press.

Horkheimer, Max. 1972. "Authority and the Family." In *Critical Theory: Selected Essays*. New York: Herder and Herder.

Hurtado, Sylvia, Mark E. Engberg, Luis Ponjuan, and Lisa Landreman. 2002. "Students' Precollege Preparation for Participation in a Diverse Democracy." *Research in Higher Education* 43 (2): 163–86.

Jeffres, Leo W., David Atkin, and Kimberly A. Neuendorf. 2002. "A Model Linking Community Activity and Communication with Political Attitudes and Involvement in Neighborhoods." *Political Communication* 19 (4): 387–421.

Jian, Guowei, and Leo Jeffres. 2008. "Spanning the Boundaries of Work: Workplace Participation, Political Efficacy, and Political Involvement." *Communication Studies* 59 (1): 35–50.

Judd, Charles Hubbard. 1918. *The Evolution of a Democratic School System*. New York: Houghton Mifflin.

Kentand Jennings, M., and Richard G. Niemi. 1981. *Generations and Politics*. Princeton: Princeton University Press.

King, Cheryl S., Camilla Stivers, and Collaborators. 1998. *Government Is Us: Public Administration in an Anti-Government Era*. Thousand Oaks, CA: Sage.

Kirlin, Mary. 2003. "The Role of Civic Skills in Fostering Civic Engagement." Working paper. College Park, MD: The Center for Information and Research on Civic Learning and Engagement.

Kjaer, Anne Mette. 2004. *Governance*. London: Polity Press.

Kohn, M. L. 1977. *Class and Conformity: A Study in Values*. Chicago: University of Chicago Press.

Kohn, M. L., and K. Schooler. 1981. "Job Conditions and Personality: A Longitudinal Assessment of Their Reciprocal Effects." In *Factor Analysis and Measurement in Sociological Research: A Multidimensional Perspective,* ed. D.J. Jackson and E.F. Borgatta. Thousand Oaks, CA: Sage.

Kumar, Sushil, Shashi Kant, and Terry L. Amburgey. 2007. "Public Agencies and Collaborative Management Approaches—Examining Resistance among Administrative Professionals." *Administration & Society* 39 (5): 569–611.

Kupchik, Aaron, and Torin Monahan. 2006. "The New American School: Preparation for Post-industrial Discipline." *British Journal of Sociology of Education* 27 (5): 617–31.

Lacey, Robert J. 2008. *American Pragmatism and Democratic Faith*. Dekalb: Northern Illinois University Press.

Lakoff, George. 2002. *Moral Politics: How Conservatives and Liberals Think*. 2nd ed. Chicago: University of Chicago Press.

Lambert, Susan J. 1990. "Processes Linking Work and Family: A Critical Review and Research Agenda." *Human Relations* 43 (3): 239–57.

Lancaster, Jane. 2004. *Making Time: Lillian Moller Gilbreth, a Life Beyond Cheaper by the Dozen.* Boston, MA: Northeastern University Press.

Lichterman, Paul. 2009. "Social Capacity and the Styles of Group Life: Some Inconvenient Wellsprings of Democracy." *American Behavioral Scientist* 52 (6): 846–66.

Mason, Ronald M. 1982. *Participatory and Workplace Democracy: A Theoretical Development in Critique of Liberalism.* Carbondale: Southern Illinois University Press.

McFarland, Daniel A., and Reuben J. Thomas. 2006. "Bowling Young: How Youth Voluntary Associations Influence Adult Political Participation." *American Journal of Sociology* 71: 401–25.

McLanahan, Sara, and Christine Percheski. 2008. "Family Structure and the Reproduction of Inequalities." *Annual Review of Sociology* 34: 257–76.

McSwite, O.C. 1997. *Legitimacy in Public Administration: A Discourse Analysis.* Thousand Oaks, CA: Sage.

———. 2005. "Taking Public Administration Seriously: Beyond Humanism and Bureaucrat Bashing." *Administration & Society* 37 (1): 116–25.

Mettler, Susan. 2002. "Bringing the State Back in to Civic Engagement: Policy Feedback Effects of the GI Bill for World War II Veterans." *American Political Science Review* 96 (2): 351–65.

Mitscherlich, Alexander. (1963) 1969. *Society without the Father: A Contribution to Social Psychology,* trans. E. Mosbacher. New York: Harcourt, Brace & World.

Pateman, Carol. 1970. *Participation and Democratic Theory.* New York: Cambridge University Press.

Perry, James L. 1997. "Antecedents of Public Service Motivation." *Journal of Public Administration Research and Theory* 7 (2): 181–97.

———. 2000. "Bringing Society In: Toward a Theory of Public-Service Motivation." *Journal of Public Administration Research and Theory* 10 (2): 471–88.

Perry, James L., and Michael C. Katula. 2001. "Does Service Affect Citizenship?" *Administration & Society* 33 (3): 330–65.

Perry, James L., and Lois Recascino Wise. 1990. "The Motivational Bases for Public Service." *Public Administration Review* 50 (3): 367–73.

Persson, Stefan, Hakan Stattin, and Margaret Kerr. 2004. "Adolescents' Conception of Family Democracy: Does Their Own Behaviour Play a Role?" *European Journal of Developmental Psychology* 1 (4): 317–30.

Putnam, Robert D. 1993. *Making Democracy Work: Civic Traditions in Modern Italy.* Princeton: Princeton University Press.

———. 2000. *Bowling Alone: The Collapse and Revival of American Community.* New York: Simon & Schuster.

Rhodes, R.A.W. 1996. "The New Governance: Governing without Government." *Political Studies* 44: 652–67.

Rimmerman, Craig A. 1997. *The New Citizenship: Unconventional Politics, Activism, and Service.* Boulder, CO: Westview Press.

Ritchie, L. David. 1997. "Parents' Workplace Experiences and Family Communication Patterns." *Communication Research* 24 (2): 175–87.

Schmidt, Mary R. 1993. "Grout: Alternative Kinds of Knowledge and Why They Are Ignored." *Public Administration Review* 53 (6): 525–30.

Schwartz, Gary. 1987. *Beyond Conformity or Rebellion: Youth and Authority in America.* Chicago: University of Chicago Press.

Staines, Graham L. 1980. "Spillover versus Compensation: A Review of the Literature on the Relationship between Work and Nonwork." *Human Relations* 33 (2): 111–29.

Stivers, Camilla. 2000. *Bureau Men, Settlement Women: Constructing Public Administration in the Progressive Era.* Lawrence: University Press of Kansas.

Stoker, Gerry. 1998. "Governance as Theory: Five Propositions." *International Social Science Journal* 50 (155): 17–28.

Verba, Sidney, Kay Lehman Schlozman, and Henry Brady. 1995. *Voice and Equality: Civic Voluntarism in American Politics.* Cambridge, MA: Harvard University Press.

Wacquant, Loïc. 2001. "The Penalisation of Poverty and the Rise of Neo-liberalism." *European Journal on Criminal Policy and Research* 9: 401–12.

———. 2002. "Slavery to Mass Incarceration: Rethinking the 'Race Question' in the U.S." *New Left Review* 13: 41–60.

Waldo, Dwight. 1948. *The Administrative State: A Study of the Political Theory of American Public Administration.* New York: Ronald Press.

White, Orion F. 1990. "Reframing the Authority Participation Debate." In *Refounding Public Administration,* ed. G.L. Wamsley et al. Newbury Park, CA: Sage.

Yang, Kaifeng. 2005. "Public Administrators' Trust in Citizens: A Missing Link in Citizen Involvement Efforts." *Public Administration Review* 65 (3): 273–85.

———. 2006. "Trust and Citizen Involvement Decisions—Trust in Citizens, Trust in Institutions, and Propensity to Trust." *Administration & Society* 38 (5): 573–95.

Yang, Kaifeng, and Kathy Callahan. 2005. "Assessing Citizen Involvement Efforts by Local Government." *Public Performance and Management Review* 29 (2): 191–216.

4

The Citizenship Role of the Public Professional

Imagining Private Lives and Alternative Futures

Richard C. Box

The Citizenship Role of the Public Professional: Imagining Private Lives and Alternative Futures

A key issue in public administration is whether public professionals should contribute to constructive change or instead serve as neutral implementers of decisions made by elected leaders. Contributing to change can involve modifying service delivery practices, making policy recommendations to decision makers, and facilitating citizen involvement in the policy-making process.

This issue is not only academic, it can be very important to the lives and work of public professionals and the people they serve. It appears in textbooks and in articles in professional magazines and scholarly journals in several forms, for example as the politics–administration relationship, administrative discretion, administrative legitimacy, customer service, and citizen involvement/participation. Broadly, it is about the extent to which public employees bear some responsibility for the condition of democracy and the outcomes of public governance.

One view on this issue is that the appropriate role of public employees is to carry out the decisions of elected officials, exercising as little interpretation or individual initiative (administrative discretion) as possible. This so-called neutrality perspective is often favored by people who prefer a clear separation of politics (the process of deciding what to do) and administration (implementing those decisions).

Another view holds that public service practitioners are important actors in public decision making, along with elected officials, individual members

60   RICHARD C. BOX

of the public, and interest groups. This perspective acknowledges that public professionals have useful knowledge and training that other actors likely do not, and that they are often closely involved in the process of providing information about current conditions and suggesting action alternatives. Though elected officials are commonly assumed to be the appropriate representatives of government to sense people's needs and preferences, many public professionals are involved in the public's lives and concerns on a daily basis and they have important knowledge that can be brought to bear in creating and implementing public policies.

These views are not mutually exclusive. At any point in time, a particular public professional may use them in different proportions depending upon the needs of the moment. In the first perspective, public professionals support the political and bureaucratic institution of government, so we may call this an *institutional public service role*. In the second perspective, they help others identify and implement solutions to public problems, which involves acting as an expert citizen, so we may call it a *citizenship public service role* (the citizenship wording follows Cooper 1991).

The institutional role can serve as a baseline, and it is what the American public traditionally expects of public employees. In contrast, the citizenship role can make people uneasy, it can stir controversy, and many public service practitioners feel uncomfortable with it even if they use it in their daily work. The citizenship role is the focus of the discussion in this chapter because we already know that a number of public employees are involved in public policy and decision-making processes, so it is important to understand how they contribute to constructive change.

Facilitating citizen involvement has long been an important and often controversial part of the citizenship role of the public professional. The first of the four sections that follow examines the concept of citizen self-governance from three perspectives: an elite perspective, a democratic perspective, and an efficiency perspective. These perspectives provide a guide for understanding the political surroundings that influence the relationship between citizens and government. Taken together, they suggest that in contemporary society it is often awkward and costly to fully involve citizens in talking about public policies and programs. This leaves open the question of what the public professional who believes in democratic, participatory government should do.

The second section of the chapter describes the status of citizen involvement today, setting it in the context of historical efforts to make governing more democratic. It shows how difficult citizen involvement can be in an environment characterized by powerful interests, an apathetic public, and the distractions of contemporary life.

These initial sections set the stage for exploring two ways that public

THE CITIZENSHIP ROLE OF THE PUBLIC PROFESSIONAL   61

professionals can take citizen interests into account, even if citizens are not directly involved in the policy discussion. The last two sections of the chapter recognize that, while citizen participation in public governance may be valued in a democratic society, it is not always feasible or desirable. This means there may be times when public professionals take on some of the responsibility for understanding public needs and interests. "Imagining private lives" suggests a way to use knowledge of current conditions that is especially helpful in the absence of public involvement, and "imagining alternative futures" describes a process for envisioning a future that is not entirely bound by the past.

These techniques are not new or unusual and many people apply them in some form to their everyday work—the purpose here is to draw attention to them and encourage their use. This discussion does not advocate particular normative ends (for example, social equity or environmental sustainability), leaving goals and values to the judgment of each public professional.

Three Perspectives on Citizen Self-Governance

Three quite different perspectives on the idea that citizens should have the opportunity to influence public policy and its implementation can be identified: an elite perspective, a democratic perspective, and an efficiency perspective. Each perspective can be traced back through time, and each can be found in the attitudes and practices of people today. To the extent a public professional emphasizes one or more of these perspectives in performing daily tasks, the preferred perspective(s) may have significant effects on the lives of people the professional serves.

The elite perspective discourages citizen involvement because the public is not considered capable of managing its own affairs, the democratic perspective argues that citizens have the right to influence actions taken by their own government, and the efficiency perspective highlights the costs in time and resources of citizen participation in decision making. The perspective that elected officials, political appointees, and public professionals emphasize in their work may make a difference in how the public is—or is not—involved in shaping public policy. In the many situations where the public is not directly involved, the question becomes how public professionals can build sensitivity to public concerns into the decision-making process.

The Elite Perspective

The contemporary question of whether Americans can and should participate in public governance beyond electing their leaders appears to echo the debate between the anti-Federalists and Federalists in the late 1780s over ratifica-

62 RICHARD C. BOX

tion of the Constitution. Fearing the public as a leveling force of democratic disorder and potential redistribution of wealth, the Federalists sought to create a national government that would be removed from everyday politics and ordinary people. This national government would be governed by "the best men in the country" (John Jay, in Quinn 1993, 20), an elite with the time and education to make rational decisions that would be "filtered," removed from the passions of the masses (Quinn 1993, 20).

Whether because of the Federalists' design for the national government or its size today, most people think they can have little influence on events at that level. The relationship between the nation and the states was a significant issue during the Founding era, and the anti-Federalists wanted to protect the powers of state governments. Local government was not at issue in the constitutional debate because it was assumed to be a creation of each state, not a matter for the national constitution, but the anti-Federalists wanted to preserve the sort of dialogue and direct connection that existed between citizens and government in small communities. Today, much of the activity in citizen involvement takes place at the local level, reflecting the realities of large-scale modern society and the concerns of the anti-Federalists.

The elite perspective on citizen involvement in governance is evident in the Federalist attitude about citizens. In 1774, Gouverneur Morris described ordinary people as the "the mob," using this language:

> I stood on the balcony and on my right hand were ranged all the people of property, with some poor dependents, and on the other the tradesmen, etc., who thought it worth their while to leave their daily labour for the good of the country. . . . The mob began to think and reason. Poor reptiles! It is with them a *vernal* morning: they are struggling to cast off their winter's slough. They bask in the sunshine, and ere noon they will bite, depend on it. (In Quinn 1993, 20)

Harsh as this may seem, it finds an echo a century later in Woodrow Wilson's well-known 1887 essay, "The Study of Administration." The essay is often assigned to students in public administration courses to illustrate early interest in a field of study and practice somewhat distinct and removed from partisan politics. Often missed is Wilson's view of the public; he finds "the bulk of mankind" to be "rigidly unphilosophical," so that "a truth must become not only plain but also commonplace before it will be seen by the people who go to their work early in the morning" (Wilson [1887] 1997, 20).

When the public becomes involved in criticizing the daily administration of government, according to Wilson, it is "a rustic handling delicate machinery"

(23). Because the people who go to their work early in the morning may vote, and public opinion can affect public policy, Wilson thought it best that an elected leader should shape public opinion, persuading people to "want the particular change he wants." To achieve this, the leader would "stir up" the public to "search for an opinion, and then manage to put the right opinion in its way" (19).

Today, the elite perspective on citizen involvement in local affairs is reflected in the belief that policy making should be left to elected leaders, or that citizen involvement must mean improper influence by a select few. It is also found in the actions of elected leaders who favor the interests of the wealthy and powerful. The story is different at the state level and especially at the national level, where the Federalist wish to separate the individual citizen from governance is more easily fulfilled. In a huge and complex arena of competing interests and elites, there is little expectation of meaningful individual influence. Broad public movements may emerge that affect the course of political affairs, and people can participate through membership in national organizations, but direct personal involvement is often limited to contributing to candidates and interest groups and voting.

The Democratic Perspective

The idea that citizens should be allowed to govern themselves is often grounded in the example of Athenian democracy, beginning in the fifth century B.C. (Lakoff 1996, chap. 3). Only a small percentage of Athenians were granted citizenship, consisting of native-born males who met certain criteria and were judged adequate by their peers. In the fifth century B.C. there may have been as many as 40,000 citizens in a total population of 250,000, which included at least 100,000 slaves. All citizens could attend and speak in the assembly, which met often to discuss a variety of issues, including selecting leaders, and decisions were made by a majority of those present (51). Though Athenians did not spell out the nature of democracy, Lakoff (1996, 60) suggests their view might have been as follows:

> Since all men are by definition capable of rationality, those who give evidence of being able to make practical use of their faculties ought to govern themselves, individually and collectively. Far from supposing that the mass of men are driven by their appetites and need to have those with reason sit on them, in Plato's image, as a rider on a horse, a democrat would contend that reason helps all people to fulfill their desires, whether these are the desires of the philosopher for comprehensive knowledge or of the ordinary man for practical wisdom and other kinds of happiness.

64   RICHARD C. BOX

So, for a relatively small group of Athenians, direct participation in public decision making was the norm, rather than a representative democracy in which elected leaders made public decisions. (Given the limited nature of citizenship in Athens, the Athenian model should be approached with caution—it illustrates the potential for exclusion and discrimination.)

The history of democratic thought in the United States can be traced through people such as Thomas Jefferson, Jane Addams, Mary Parker Follett, and John Dewey, all of whom in their own way wanted to give people the knowledge and access to public decision making they needed to take an active part in public sector governance. Thomas Jefferson wanted to add a fourth level to the trilogy of national, state, and local government. This was the "ward-republic," a subdivision of the county, in which approximately one hundred citizens would meet to discuss and vote upon matters affecting the ward and also matters related to levels of government above them, passing along their views to government at the county level, where they would be aggregated and passed to the state level, and so on.

The concept of ward-republics shows the influence of "Greek conceptions of politics and citizenship" (Matthews 1984, 83) and also Jefferson's interest in the governance system used by Native Americans (148n18). Jefferson (in a letter to Joseph C. Cabell dated February 2, 1816) wrote that the wards would give each person an opportunity to be directly involved in self-governance, so that,

> where every man is a sharer in the direction of his ward-republic, or of some of the higher ones, and feels that he is a participator in the government of affairs, not merely at an election one day in the year, but every day; when there shall not be a man in the State who will not be a member of some one of its councils, great or small, he will let the heart be torn out of his body sooner than his power be wrested from him by a Cæsar or a Bonaparte. (Jefferson [1816] 1984, 1380)

Ward-republics did not become a formal part of the system of government, but we can find their outline in today's neighborhood organizations (Box and Musso 2004). Self-governance can seem out of date in an age of electronic communities, a cynical or apathetic public, and complex, large-scale urban society, but many people still think that democracy can include direct citizen access to policy making, at least at the subnational level. Athenians believed that participating in public governance was an essential part of a fulfilling life. In contemporary society it is impractical to think that public participation will be part of everyone's life and we expect governments to do their work without constant attention from citizens. Nevertheless, the idea that people "own" their government and should have a direct voice in governance if they choose to exercise it remains important.

The Efficiency Perspective

The influence of marketlike, economistic thought began to increase in the American public sector in the 1980s, and the trend accelerated through the 1990s. Deregulation, privatization, contracting out, devolution/decentralization, and slogans such as "government is the problem, not the solution," "reinventing government," and "running government like a business" became the order of the day (Box 1999).

In a capitalist society, government is not separate from, nor immune to, the desire for efficiency, nor would we expect it to be. The relevant question "is whether economics should be the primary reason for public action, or instead one reason among several and a useful tool for carrying out policies created for other reasons" (Box 2008, 56). The societal phenomenon that currently frames the penetration of economistic thought into the public sector is "neoliberalism." The "liberalism" part of this term "refers to economic rather than political liberalism," thus to a free-market, limited-government ideology. Application of neoliberalism in the public sector "produces governance criteria ... of productivity and profitability, with the consequence that governance talk increasingly becomes market-speak" (Brown 2006, 694).

In public administration, the neoliberal emphasis on economic rationality has taken form in "new public management" and related concepts, with accompanying stress on quantification of performance and measurement of whatever can be measured. A recent extension of the idea of decentering government can be found in the concepts of "networks" and "new governance." Bingham, Nabatchi, and O'Leary (2005, 547) describe this as including "horizontal networks of public, private, and nonprofit organizations ... as opposed to hierarchical organizational decision making," and also "the citizenry—the tool makers and tool users—and the processes through which they participate in the work of government."

New governance can be thought of as part of the neoliberal agenda, weakening government's capacity to limit private sector excesses and soften the social injustice, inequality, and environmental impacts these excesses create. Alternatively, it may be regarded as a democratic influence, a way for citizens to have an effect on policy makers and bureaucracies that have resisted input from outsiders. Either way, it is reasonable to question the extent to which new governance is new or real, and to what parts of the public sector it might apply.

Certainly, contracting out public services to the nonprofit and private sectors

66   RICHARD C. BOX

and the growth of the nonprofit sector have meant changes in administrative practices and decision making, and growth in interest groups and Internet-based activity has made it possible for many more people to participate, if rather indirectly, in aspects of governance. However, contracting, distributed centers of decision making, citizen involvement, and interest groups are hardly new phenomena. These have been features of everyday practice and research for decades, especially for practitioners and academicians who focus on local government (Box 2008, 7–9).

So, the question is not whether government has suddenly changed into something different, but instead how public professionals might respond to heightened attention to economic efficiency and decision making that involves multiple groups and citizens. Efficiency in itself is not a bad thing, but it can be troublesome when it becomes an end rather than a means, displacing consideration of other important ideas, such as "constitutionalism and law, citizen self-governance, the role of the individual public service practitioner in a democratic society, the public good, and social equity" (Box 2007, 194). To the extent that public professionals respond to multiple demands by focusing on reduced cost and measurement to the exclusion of these broader matters, public governance loses a significant voice for constructive change.

In years of teaching graduate public administration students (the majority of whom are already professionals in government and the nonprofit sector), this author has found that many, if not most, are skeptical about the idea that citizens might take part in public decision making beyond the act of voting, or that they have the capacity to understand complex public issues. For some students, this skepticism is based on experience. They have witnessed people refusing to participate in community dialogue when given an opportunity and people pushing their own interests to the exclusion of others. Some students find that conducting a citizen involvement process takes more time and energy than the results merit.

Some other students have simply never been exposed to the idea of participatory democracy; they only know about the representative model of voting for elected officials who make decisions, and they cannot imagine anything different. When these students are shown a participatory model of, for example, active issue identification, prioritization, and goal setting by citizens in the budgeting process of a good-size city, they are startled to discover that democracy can mean more than voting. Given the application in public agencies nationwide of well-known citizen involvement techniques, this lack of awareness on the part of people studying public administration is remarkable.

The extent to which economic rationality affects scholarly views of citizen involvement is illustrated in a *Public Administration Review* article (Irvin and Stansbury 2004) titled "Citizen Participation in Decision Making: Is It Worth the Effort?" As the title implies, the authors challenge the assumption that citizen participation is good in itself, and suggest ways that practitioners can determine whether it will be cost-effective in time and resources. Citizen involvement is treated here as a technique that public managers may choose to employ after they apply the authors' "litmus test for agencies to consider when they allocate resources for citizen-participation processes" (62). Before neoliberalism became a pervasive societal context for the public sector, we might have expected some public professionals to assume, at least at the local level, that citizens are the "owners" of their government and thus have the right to participate as they wish. If this prescriptive litmus test is followed, the public will or will not be involved depending on whether an efficiency-conscious administrator determines it does not cost too much.

The criteria given by Irvin and Stansbury for deciding whether citizen participation is cost-effective seem reasonable and practical. The authors emphasize citizen participation processes created for one-time needs rather than those that are permanently integrated into agencies, but their argument for attention to resource allocation makes sense—citizen involvement is not always useful, and public resources are limited.

It can be argued that a central purpose of democratic government is to involve the public in governance, and that cost-effectiveness should not be the primary factor that determines whether decision making includes citizens. However, given the influence in American society of the elite perspective and the realities of limited resources and a public not much interested in direct involvement, the economic perspective is important.

Current Conditions in Citizen Involvement

Citizen involvement may be thought of as a recent phenomenon that arose in the social turmoil and concern for citizen empowerment in the 1960s, grew dramatically in public awareness and application in government at all levels in the 1970s, and leveled off beginning with the reign of Reaganite conservatives in the 1980s. However, the relationship between citizens and government is as old as government and politics, and in the United States it began in the Colonial era. It was especially prominent in the debate over the ratification of the Constitution, as the anti-Federalists argued that the Federalists wanted to shift power and wealth from the states and ordinary people to a national government and the elite (Wood 1969). (For our purposes here, citizen involvement or participation is defined as residents taking part in public decision-making processes beyond those of traditional bodies such as planning or parks commissions.)

68   RICHARD C. BOX

During the nineteenth century, property qualifications for voting were lifted, Jeffersonian and Jacksonian democracy at the national level moved away from the idea of government run by the wealthy and wise, and in local governments a variety of structures and practices developed that allowed people to participate in policy making and supervision of administration (Box 1998). Toward the end of the nineteenth century and into the early twentieth century, two related trends were at work. One was reforms intended to strengthen leadership so that government would be more efficient, such as introduction of the strong-mayor, commission, and council-manager forms of city government. This trend ran counter to the democratizing impulse of the nineteenth century, though it can be argued that it helped rescue democracy from the corruption of urban machines. The other trend was the Progressive-era desire of people to participate directly in public affairs. In cities, the community centers movement exemplified this desire, as people gathered together, often in school buildings, to discuss and debate current issues of importance (Mattson 1998).

With the exception of established practices in some local areas, the impulse toward citizen involvement in public governance lost energy from the 1920s through the 1950s. The Progressive-era wish for social change had faded by the end of World War I and into the 1920s. The Great Depression, World War II, and the immediate postwar period were times in which government grew and became professionalized, with bureaucratic systems and maximization of efficiency rather than direct democracy.

This brings us back to the 1960s. During the 1960s and 1970s there were a number of national government programs that included mandates for citizen involvement, but many of them were discontinued during the Reagan administration in the 1980s on grounds that they were part of a "liberal agenda" (Berry, Portney, and Thomson 1993, chap. 2). Meanwhile, state and local citizen involvement programs grew during this period and, in some places and with varying degrees of success, they continue to grow and thrive today. The land-use planning system in Oregon, begun in 1973, is an example of a statewide mandate for citizen involvement in local government (Oregon Department of Land Conservation and Development 2010). Some local governments have relatively informal citizen involvement processes in which staff and elected officials may interact with residents periodically in relation to projects, budgeting, or local issues. Others have programs staffed by local government professionals in which residents become continuing partners in decision making, such as the priority boards in Dayton, Ohio (City of Dayton, Ohio, 2010). Some, such as the City of Seattle, show an emphasis on neighborhoods in the structure of local government (City of Seattle, Washington, 2010); among other measures, Seattle has created "service centers" to geographically decentralize city departments. A number of citizen involvement initiatives emphasize particular governmental functions, such as planning, budgeting (Franklin and Ebdon 2007), and performance measurement (Ho 2007).

If it were easy to participate meaningfully in creating and implementing public policy, it is likely that many people would want to take part. However, in most places and at most times it is not easy, but instead takes considerable time and effort. Sometimes this is just because democracy is messy and complex, so that people have to work through gathering information and understanding the issues, listening to and appreciating the ideas and interests of others, and crafting solutions. Often, though, participation is not easy because there are barriers such as complicated legal requirements, bureaucratic systems, poorly designed involvement programs that allow special interests to dominate, the influence of wealthy and powerful people who use government to advance their financial interests, and public professionals who find citizen involvement disruptive or inefficient (Box, Marshall, Reed, and Reed 2001; Box and Sagen 1998; King, Feltey, and Susel 1998). Supposedly participatory processes can instead be opportunities for governing bodies to tell the public what they have already decided or for residents, groups, public agency staff, or private firms with particular interests to influence decisions. A largely apathetic citizenry might stay at home, unaware of the issues, busy with other things, or thinking that their input would make little difference.

Apathy, cynicism, and mistrust toward government are not new (Nye, Zelikow, and King 1997). It has always been true that many people know little about the public sector and do not care about it, some know about it but are not interested in being personally involved, and some actively dislike it because of perceived corruption, ineffectiveness, special-interest control, or some other dysfunction. This leaves some of those most directly affected by government actions and a small percentage of the general citizenry to participate in making public policy and supervising its implementation.

In addition to the apathy and cynicism that have always been present, the contemporary societal setting includes a range of pressures and distractions that may make meaningful citizen participation even more difficult and unlikely than in earlier times. As others have noted (Bennett 1998; Putnam 2000), electronic viewing and communications (television, the Internet, cell phones, etc.) occupy an increasing portion of people's lives, plus economic conditions are pushing people into spending more time in activities directly related to making a living. Contributing to the well-being of society by taking part in public affairs (beyond the act of voting) is not a priority for many people, a circumstance that seems unlikely to change in the near future.

70   RICHARD C. BOX

Imagining Private Lives

The picture of citizen self-governance painted here is mixed. It includes some units of government in which the public has significant opportunities to influence public policy, it includes in some places resistance to an open decision-making process by powerful elites or administrators who dislike perceived intrusion into their activities, and it includes in many times and places a public relatively indifferent toward public affairs. Where citizen involvement processes are used, they may be permanent (such as neighborhood groups or advisory bodies) or they may exist for a limited time to address a specific need. They may share considerable decision-making responsibility with their host government or serve largely to promote dialogue and communication, and they may have substantial staff support from public professionals or operate on their own.

This mixed picture leaves open the question of what a public professional might do in times and places where direct citizen involvement is impractical or unlikely. If this professional thinks that the diverse wishes and preferences of citizens should somehow be taken into account, she or he may try "imagining private lives." This is not a new idea and many people already do it—the point here is to give the technique a name and to encourage its use.

In places where citizen involvement is often a part of decision making, there may be a culture of shared responsibility for public policy and governance. In the more common setting of programs or units of government where citizen involvement is not generally used, it is often assumed that elected officials will represent the interests of the public, searching for some approximation of what the majority of people think is best ("the public interest").

This raises the question of whether elected governing bodies fairly represent the interests of all the residents in a government's jurisdiction. Some governing bodies seem to do this well, but some seem inept at dealing with complex public issues, and some others appear intent on serving mostly the interests of prominent or active citizens. There is often value in having public professionals take part in the process of sensing public needs and suggesting policy options (Box 2008, chap. 3), but it can be even more important when this "political failure" occurs.

Public professionals who choose to take part in constructive change can do so from the position of "the citizen who is employed *as* one of us to work *for* us; a kind of professional citizen ordained to do that work which we in a complex large-scale political community are unable to undertake ourselves" (Cooper 1991, 139). They can "imagine private lives" (Box 2005, chap. 6), that is, they can use what they know of physical, economic, and social conditions to fashion recommendations and operating procedures that serve particular ends.

THE CITIZENSHIP ROLE OF THE PUBLIC PROFESSIONAL   71

Imagining conditions in the social and physical environment is not an act of vague emotionalism, it is a matter of assembling knowledge gained through working with projects, problems, and conditions in the everyday work setting. Thanks to training and experience, public professionals are able to describe and interpret this knowledge in ways that would be difficult for others. The issues and conditions they describe may need immediate attention, such as a significant increase in violence and street shootings, pollution of a major waterway, or deteriorating highway bridges. They can also be things that are not so pressing but are equally important, for example streetscape designs that do not address the needs of the elderly and disabled, overuse of forests or fisheries, or inadequate health care or education for a minority population.

Public sector employees work in a wide range of occupational specializations and as a group they have a large and varied set of normative preferences for constructive change. (For discussion of the normative ends valued by public service practitioners, see Box 1998, chap. 5; 2007; 2008, chap. 3; Van Wart 1998.) Social workers, intelligence officers, land use planners, housing program managers, and so on have interests and concerns that are specific to their fields of practice. How they apply their preferences for change can be strongly influenced by the political, economic, and social circumstances of the places in which they work (Box 1998, chap. 2).

Public professionals working within the citizenship role can use the technique of imagining private lives to assist them in offering policy ideas to residents and elected decision makers. They can also use it to analyze service delivery and make changes that will advance the normative ends they value. This need not mean violating the expectations that elected officials and the public have for the role of the public professional. It means that everyday decisions about resource allocation and service delivery can be informed by awareness of the things people care about and the effects of one's actions on their lives. For example, one might ask: Could we make residents feel safer from street violence by changing our patrol strategy? Can we increase successful outcomes with social services clients by focusing on individual circumstances rather than rules and processes? Are we doing enough to protect forest lands for the use and enjoyment of people today and those in future generations?

Imagining Alternative Futures

Identifying and implementing appropriate policies and programs can be challenging in a society with diverse interests. Feldman and Khademian (2007) describe three perspectives on public policy: the political, technical, and experiential, corresponding to elected leaders, public professionals, and citizens. The authors suggest that "bringing people together from different perspectives in ways that allow them to appreciate one another's perspectives will enhance the design as well as implementation of policies" (306).

From within each of these perspectives, though, it can be difficult for people to think about the perspectives of others and ways the future could be different from the present. We can become so accustomed to the way things seem to us, to how politics, economics, and organizations function today, that envisioning something different can be annoying or even threatening. This phenomenon can operate at a macro level, for example with views about war and international affairs, or it can operate on a smaller scale, for example with views on growth management in an urban area.

Whatever the scale, it can be difficult to recognize there are multiple ways of thinking about an issue that are different from one's own. This difficulty can be reinforced by the media, popular opinion, and organizational dogma, which often reflect the dominant views of the powerful and act to limit questioning and critique (Marcuse 1964). A national-level example from recent history would be the time just before and during the early stages of the war in Iraq. A local example could be political pressure exerted to promote the idea of rapid growth and expansion, despite potential environmental impacts. People who question a dominant view may experience criticism, ridicule, or negative career impacts, which may encourage others to avoid these consequences by ignoring possible alternatives.

Imagining alternative futures is an effective way to encourage thinking beyond what is likely to occur if present circumstances continue unchanged into the future. It offers people the opportunity to consciously shape future conditions rather than waiting for them to happen. This is not an unusual or exotic technique; it can be found in scenario planning (Ogilvy 2002) and it is a common tool in land-use planning (Hoch 2000). As an example found in many communities, planners and local residents may be concerned about the rate, form, cost, and environmental impacts of physical growth in housing and commercial land use. They may choose to imagine the effects of alternative approaches to these issues as a way to select preferred policies for the future.

There are a number of techniques being used in local governments to manage growth and minimize negative impacts, but residents and elected leaders may not be aware of them. This means it is left to planners, public professionals, to assemble data on local growth, gather information on growth management practices in other places, and show several alternative futures for the community that depend on possible policy actions. The alternative futures might show projected conditions related to traffic flows, costs of providing infrastructure, air pollution, social conditions in the central city, and so on.

THE CITIZENSHIP ROLE OF THE PUBLIC PROFESSIONAL   73

Rather than present their work in a "public hearing," which could pit people concerned about the living environment against people who think of the community as a place to make money, planners might work with committees of volunteers and in open neighborhood workshops, taking care to be inclusive and to avoid over-representation by those with predetermined agendas. This gives many residents opportunities to understand current reality, the perspectives of others, and alternative ways the community might develop.

If this process goes well, when it is complete the city council might create an ongoing volunteer board (with specified duties, membership, and professional staff support) to work with the existing planning commission, offering periodic assessment of urban growth planning. In this way, imagining alternative futures and evaluating implementation over time become a permanent part of how the community thinks about its physical form, economy, social conditions, environmental sustainability, and aesthetics.

By using examples of practices from other places and open discussion of alternative futures, the community can avoid status quo thinking that thoughtlessly replicates present circumstances instead of consciously choosing a desired future. This example sets the technique of imagining alternative futures in the context of citizen involvement. However, it can also be applied effectively in settings where only professionals, or professionals and elected leaders, assess current conditions and plan for future actions.

Conclusion

The discussion in this chapter describes mixed experience with public involvement. There are examples of successful citizen participation in policy making, and there are also challenges to involvement posed by the complexity of government, resistance from those with something to lose and administrators who dislike "interference," and a public that has competing time demands or that may be apathetic. Though these challenges are significant, there is a need for informed decision making and government that serves not only the interests of the powerful but also the broader public.

Because public professionals have knowledge and skills that other public sector actors often do not, they have opportunities to create constructive change through service delivery practices and by offering knowledge and assistance to elected leaders and citizens. Sometimes this may be accomplished by working with the public, but often it is a matter of working within the organization and offering advice to elected leaders.

Public professionals can use the techniques of imagining private lives and imagining alternative futures to improve the fit between public services and public needs and to expand the range of possibilities beyond the way things

74   RICHARD C. BOX

are today. Serving in the citizenship role is not appropriate for everyone nor is it useful in all times and places, and it carries risks that the institutional role does not. One source of risk is the displeasure of people who think their interests are threatened by open discussion of alternatives. Another is the potential for public professionals to violate the expectations their organizational peers, elected officials, or the public have for the role of the public professional. Despite the difficulties and risks, imagining private lives and imagining alternative futures are effective tools for public professionals who wish to contribute to constructive change.

References

Bennett, W. Lance. 1998. "The Uncivic Culture: Communication, Identity, and the Rise of Lifestyle Politics." *Political Science & Politics* 31 (4): 741–61.

Berry, Jeffrey M., Kent E. Portney, and Ken Thomson. 1993. *The Rebirth of Urban Democracy.* Washington, DC: Brookings Institution Press.

Bingham, Lisa B., Tina Nabatchi, and Rosemary O'Leary. 2005. "The New Governance: Practices and Processes for Stakeholder and Citizen Participation in the Work of Government." *Public Administration Review* 65 (5): 547–58.

Box, Richard C. 1998. *Citizen Governance: Leading American Communities into the 21st Century.* Thousand Oaks, CA: Sage.

———. 1999. "Running Government Like a Business: Implications for Public Administration Theory and Practice." *American Review of Public Administration* 29 (1): 19–43.

———. 2005. *Critical Social Theory in Public Administration.* Armonk, NY: M.E. Sharpe.

———. 2007. "The Public Service Practitioner as Agent of Social Change. In *Democracy and Public Administration,* ed. Richard C. Box. Armonk, NY: M.E. Sharpe.

———. 2008. *Making a Difference: Progressive Values in Public Administration.* Armonk, NY: M.E. Sharpe.

Box, Richard C., Gary S. Marshall, B.J. Reed, and Cristine M. Reed. 2001. "New Public Management and Substantive Democracy." *Public Administration Review* 61 (5): 608–19.

Box, Richard C., and Juliet A. Musso. 2004. "Experiments with Local Federalism: Secession and the Neighborhood Council Movement in Los Angeles." *American Review of Public Administration* 34 (3): 259–76.

Box, Richard C., and Deborah A. Sagen. 1998. "Working with Citizens: Breaking Down Barriers to Citizen Self-governance." In *Government Is Us: Public Administration in an Anti-Government Era,* ed. Cheryl Simrell King and Camilla Stivers. Thousand Oaks, CA: Sage.

Brown, Wendy. 2006. "American Nightmare: Neoliberalism, Neoconservatism, and De-democratization." *Political Theory* 34 (6): 690–714.

City of Dayton, Ohio. 2010. "Planning and Community Development: Priority Boards." City of Dayton.org. Available at http://www.cityofdayton.org/departments/pcd/cp/Pages/PriorityBoards.aspx, accessed November 18, 2010.

City of Seattle, Washington. 2010. "Department of Neighborhoods." Seattle.gov. Available at http://www.seattle.gov/neighborhoods, accessed November 18, 2010.

Cooper, Terry L. 1991. *An Ethic of Citizenship for Public Administration.* Englewood Cliffs, NJ: Prentice Hall.

Feldman, Martha S., and Anne M. Khademian. 2007. "The Role of the Public Manager in Inclusion: Creating Communities of Participation." *Governance: An International Journal of Policy, Administration, and Institutions* 20 (2): 305–24.

Franklin, Aimee L., and Carol Ebdon. 2007. "Democracy, Public Participation, and Budgeting: Mutually Exclusive or Just Exhausting?" In *Democracy and Public Administration,* ed. Richard C. Box. Armonk, NY: M.E. Sharpe.

Ho, Alfred T. 2007. "Citizen Participation in Performance Measurement." In *Democracy and Public Administration,* ed. Richard C. Box. Armonk, NY: M.E. Sharpe.

Hoch, Charles J. 2000. "Making Plans." In *The Practice of Local Government Planning,* ed. Charles J. Hoch, Linda C. Dalton, and Frank S. So. Washington, DC: The International City/County Management Association.

Irvin, Renee A., and John Stansbury. 2004. "Citizen Participation in Decision Making: Is It Worth the Effort?" *Public Administration Review* 64 (1): 55–65.

Jefferson, Thomas. (1816) 1984. "Letter to Joseph C. Cabell." In *Thomas Jefferson, Writings,* 1377–1381. New York: The Library of America.

King, Cheryl Simrell, Kathryn M. Feltey, and Bridget O'Neill Susel. 1998. "The Question of Participation: Toward Authentic Public Participation in Public Administration." *Public Administration Review* 58 (4): 317–26.

Lakoff, Sanford. 1996. *Democracy: History, Theory, Practice.* Boulder, CO: Westview Press.

Marcuse, Herbert. 1964. *One-Dimensional Man.* Boston: Beacon Press.

Matthews, Richard K. 1984. *The Radical Politics of Thomas Jefferson: A Revisionist View.* Lawrence: University Press of Kansas.

Mattson, Kevin. 1998. *Creating a Democratic Republic: The Struggle for Urban Participatory Democracy during the Progressive Era.* University Park: Pennsylvania State University Press.

Nye, Joseph S. Jr., Philip D. Zelikow, and David C. King, ed. 1997. *Why People Don't Trust Government.* Cambridge, MA: Harvard University Press.

Ogilvy, James A. 2002. *Creating Better Futures: Scenario Planning As a Tool for a Better Tomorrow.* New York: Oxford University Press.

Oregon Department of Land Conservation and Development. 2010. "Welcome to the Department of Land Conservation and Development." Oregon.gov. Available at http://www.oregon.gov/LCD/index.shtml, accessed November 18, 2010.

Putnam, Robert D. 2000. *Bowling Alone: The Collapse and Revival of American Community.* New York: Simon & Schuster.

Quinn, Frederick, ed. 1993. *The Federalist Papers Reader.* Washington, DC: Seven Locks Press.

Van Wart, Montgomery. 1998. *Changing Public Sector Values.* New York: Garland Publishing.

Wood, Gordon S. 1969. *The Creation of the American Republic, 1776–1787.* Chapel Hill: University of North Carolina Press.

Wilson, Woodrow. (1887) 1997. "The Study of Administration." In *Classics of Public Administration,* 4th ed., ed. Jay M. Shaftiz and Albert C. Hyde. Fort Worth, TX: Harcourt Brace College.

5

Cultivating and Sustaining Empathy as a Normative Value in Public Administration

Lisa A. Zanetti

There are many respects in which America, if it can bring itself to act with the magnanimity and the empathy appropriate to its size and power, can be an intelligent example to the world.
—J. William Fulbright

Abandonment of the rules produces monsters; so does neglect of the person.
—John Noonan

Empathy is the most radical of human emotions.
—Gloria Steinem

Micrology: The interplay between the analytic and the subjective-personal; an explicit acknowledgement in multiple discourses of the need for a counterbalance to abstracted, aggregated, generalized data. See also Barthes' punctum, Bakhtin's chronotope, Derrida's concept of the trace, and Adorno's focus on the concrete particular as examples of this concern. Self-reflexivity in this manner is part of the feminist critique against objectivity and distance. Choosing certain texts, details, or situations is a political act in that it declares not only that these elements are worth studying, but openly declares one's commitment to them. Such a declaration of solidarity is part of the ethic of critical theory as well.

—Janet Wolff (1995)

This past year I was diagnosed with cancer. As *New York Times* columnist Nicholas Kristof (2010) noted in a column that appeared at roughly the same time as my own diagnosis, 41 percent of Americans now are diagnosed with some form of cancer. As with many cancer patients, the diagnosis came suddenly and treatment followed swiftly.

I have become a bit reclusive in recent years for a variety of reasons. As a natural introvert I find I can go days with no one's company but my own. I live half a continent from family and am now an empty nester, with my children living in different states. I hate to talk on the phone and rely primarily on e-mail and texting to stay in touch with loved ones. In the chaotic days immediately following my diagnosis, as we attempted to refine treatment options and set a date for surgery (a moving target), I silently blessed the variety of technology and social networking media that made it possible to spread the word quickly to friends and family as I put away my "normal" life and prepared to enter the white, quietly sterile halls of oncology.

Interestingly, although I knew I might need temporary help after the surgery, I was a bit puzzled by my friends' and family's insistence that someone be with me in the days beforehand. I was already on sabbatical, so covering my classes was not an issue, and I knew my university colleagues would not be inconvenienced by my absence. I failed to understand why anyone needed to accompany me to the hospital the morning of my surgery (I took a taxi) or wait hours in the hospital until I was out of recovery (though several friends came by my hospital room after I was released from recovery, and we shared a good dose of gallows humor). Nor would I allow family members to disrupt a planned holiday to come to Missouri to sit with me in the hospital for nearly a week until I was discharged.

In short, as a true American, I was being a stubborn individualist. The cancer was my "problem," and I would deal with it on my own to the greatest extent possible. I even contemplated, for a short time, coping on my own after release from the hospital.

I was taken aback by the vehemence with which this plan was rejected by family and friends who refused to allow me to cope on my own. One sister put work and family on hold to be there for my discharge and the days immediately following. While she was there she not only looked after me but stocked the refrigerator, freezer, and cupboards, got the house cleaned, and made sure a fallen gutter was repaired before I returned home. Colleague and friend, Cheryl Simrell King, flew to Missouri for an entire week to change bandages, cook delicious, nutritious food to tempt a nonexistent appetite, and even befriend my tribe of quirky housebound and feral cats. My parents flew out for nearly ten days and then, after the surgeon's permission, took me back to Virginia with them to recuperate for several more weeks. In between these caregivers' visits, other friends, colleagues, and a former student or two dropped by to keep me company, bring meals, fetch prescriptions, and generally provide great moral support.

Amid the many well wishes I received was one that I found particularly touching. It was from a particular group of "virtual" friends with whom I've

78   LISA A. ZANETTI

been chatting online for over two years. I shared the news of my diagnosis and told them I'd be out of touch for a while. A few days later a lovely, handmade, most nonvirtual card arrived with messages of strength and encouragement from each of them. It was a striking example of, essentially, the kindness of strangers, resonating strongly with the work I'd been doing all year on empathy and disaster situations. It caused me to ask all over again: What makes us empathize with certain people or situations over others?

Empathy: Its Cultivation and Care

Many cancer survivors echo disaster survivors as they speak emotionally of the kindnesses experienced during their time of need. Asked to give an off-the-cuff definition of empathy, most of us would say it is the ability to identify with another individual and, as Bill Clinton famously said, "feel your pain." Over the past ten years there has been increased popular and scholarly interest in the concept and the practice of empathy. Obama emphasized the concept in his book *The Audacity of Hope* (2008). Scholarship on care-centered ethics has been foundational in reorienting the discourse of moral theory (Gilligan [1982] 1993; Noddings 2002). Goleman's ([1995] 1997) best-selling book on emotional intelligence identified empathy as a critical human value. Ackerman's (2004) work focused on the possible biological origins of empathy. Pink (2006) argues the future belongs to right-brain thinkers and names empathy as one of the "six new senses."

Why focus on empathy in a book about public administration? The enduring importance of empathy emerges from its inevitable connection to social organization. Hoffman (2000) writes of empathy: "*it epitomizes the existential human dilemma of how people come to grips with the inevitable conflicts between their egoistic needs and their social obligations*" (1–2, emphasis mine). Empathy appears to have a strong evolutionary foundation; many mammals experience empathy to some degree, particularly social animals, as empathy helps them read one another and figure out how to act. In its simplest form, empathy is observed in mirroring actions (Ackerman 2004). Evidence is accumulating that this mechanism is ancient, probably as old as mammals and birds.

But more important for the argument here is the evidence that humans tend to be most empathetic with those they perceive to be most like themselves. Batson and colleagues (2002) looked at three stigmatized groups: AIDS patients, the homeless, and violent criminals. In the first study, female participants felt more empathy for a young woman with AIDS when they were asked to take her perspective rather than be objective. This effect was lessened, however, when they were led to believe the young woman was responsible for having contracted AIDS. In addition, feelings of empathy led to better attitudes toward people with AIDS, except when the target group was extremely similar to the participants (young women) and responsible for having AIDS.

A second experiment looked at a more stigmatized group: the homeless. Feelings of empathy for a homeless man increased attitudes for the homeless in general. Again, responsibility of the homeless man for his condition lessened feelings of empathy. Finally, the third study used convicted murderers as the target group. Short-term laboratory results showed that empathetic feelings were related to more favorable attitudes toward murderers. A week later, a telephone interviewer called participants and asked about their attitudes toward prison reform. Attitudes were more favorable when participants were induced to feel more empathy towards a killer (Batson et al. 2002).

Even more revealing is the latest research on empathy coming to us from the field of neuroscience. Research conducted by social neuroscientists at the University of Toronto at Scarborough explored the sensitivity of the "mirror-neuron-system" to race and ethnicity. The researchers had study participants view a series of videos while hooked up to electroencephalogram (EEG) machines. The participants—all white—watched simple videos in which men of different races picked up a glass and took a sip of water. They watched white, black, South Asian, and East Asian men perform the task. Researchers found that there is a basic difference in the way peoples' brains react to those from other ethnic backgrounds. Observing someone of a different race produced significantly less motor-cortex activity than observing a person of one's own race. In other words, people were less likely mentally to simulate the actions of other-race than same-race people (Gutsell and Inzlicht 2010).

In other words, *empathy for those we perceive as unlike ourselves must be actively cultivated and sustained.* Our brains must be trained to experience empathy for out-group members. It's not an evolutionarily conditioned reflex. This, to me, suggests disturbing implications for the public sphere that I discuss further on.

"Trying to Reason with Hurricane Season": Jimmy Buffett

As a child in a military family I lived in many places, but the family ultimately settled in the Hampton Roads, Virginia, region (formerly known as Tidewater). The occasional hurricane is a fact of life, but concern has been higher since Hurricane Isabel clobbered the state in 2003, and, of course, since New Orleans's disastrous evacuation experience with Hurricane Katrina in 2005.

Typically, the average resident in Hampton Roads (which, geographically, runs seamlessly into the Outer Banks of North Carolina) opts for the "rugged individualist" approach to hurricanes: stock up on water, batteries, and

80   LISA A. ZANETTI

canned goods; fill the car with gas; put the patio furniture in the pool so the wind doesn't blow it through the sliding glass windows; have ice and coolers on hand to salvage the refrigerator contents if the power goes out; and maybe board up the windows if it looks like it's going to be a strong one. Those who've lived through a hurricane or two may have a back-up generator, wind and flood vents on the house, and extra insurance. Then sit back, mix up some margaritas, and throw a hurricane party. What else can you do? Nature has a mind of its own.

Compared to the Gulf Coast or the Carolinas, the Virginia coast historically hasn't had as much to worry about when it comes to hurricanes. The fortuitous combination of geography and cooler waters mean the area hasn't had a direct hit since Tropical Storm Danielle in 1992. Still, a recent report listed Miami, Florida, and Virginia Beach, Virginia, as the two cities most at risk for residential damage from storm surge if hit directly by a Category 5 hurricane, predicting damage in Virginia Beach alone to the tune of $39 billion and some 250,000 properties. Those figures account only for damage to structures, not vehicles, furniture, and other household contents. Furthermore, because of the region's jagged coastline and extensive bridge-and-tunnel network, an inland evacuation avoiding those structures could take more than 36 hours and still leave many residents stranded. In other words, the region is very vulnerable.

I mention these alarming statistics as a comparison to the City of New Orleans and its experience with Hurricane Katrina. Hampton Roads is a smaller area geographically than New Orleans—2,647 square miles compared to 4,190 square miles for New Orleans—but has a larger population. Estimates for the 2010 census range as high as two million, compared to the 1.3 million population of New Orleans in 2005, before Katrina. Hampton Roads has a much denser population, features ten cities, six counties, and one town; and multiple military installations for the U.S. Navy, Army, Air Force, Marines, NASA, and Coast Guard. The region sits entirely at sea level and is steeped in 400 years of American history, including artifacts of the nation's first landing at Jamestown in 1607 and the nation's second-oldest institution of higher education, the College of William & Mary, founded in 1693. Surely, evacuating such an area would be at least as challenging as was evacuating New Orleans.

Many observers blamed the City of New Orleans for not issuing evacuation orders earlier and for not evacuating the city more efficiently. But, like residents of Hampton Roads, many New Orleanians historically took a ruggedly individualistic approach to hurricanes, figuring that if they had survived Hurricane Camille in 1969 they had earned their stripes, so to speak. By the time the National Hurricane Center knew on August 27, 2005, that Katrina

CULTIVATING AND SUSTAINING EMPATHY AS A NORMATIVE VALUE   81

was strengthening and heading straight for New Orleans and had a mandatory evacuation order issued on August 28, it was too late to effectively evacuate the city, especially the least mobile citizens.

It's not as if these cities don't try to be prepared. Community emergency management (disaster preparedness) has moved to center stage in the past decade or so. Comprehensive emergency management first emerged in 1979 from the National Governor's Association as jurisdictions began to recognize the complexity and diversity of possible hazards. Mitigation, preparedness, and response and recovery activities had to be coordinated among actors in the public, private, and nonprofit sectors. By focusing too much on specific hazards, however, this approach failed to recognize the social, political, economic, cultural, and other variables that contribute to a disaster scenario (McEntire, Fuller, Johnston, and Weber 2002).

Next, emergency planners tried to move to creating "disaster-resistant communities" (Geis 2000). This involved assisting communities in minimizing their vulnerability to natural hazards. Hazard and vulnerability analyses, prezoning methods, land-use planning, community education, and more stringent building codes and regulations were implemented. Community grants were available through the Federal Emergency Management Agency's Project Impact program. Still, this approach tended to focus only on extreme natural disaster events and did not attempt to assess social, civil, and technological triggering agents or include emergency managers, meteorologists, first responders, hazmat teams, public health officials, or the nonprofit sector. Nor did it address how constraining attitudes, psychological stress, and political processes relate to disaster (McEntire et al. 2002).

The "disaster-resilient community" approach focuses on resilience as a measure of a community's ability to recover after a disaster. Prevention of disaster may not always be possible, and this approach acknowledges that different communities will not respond or recover in the same way. Higher levels of resilience (determined by assessing a community's economic, psychological, and cultural indicators) would suggest a reduced need for assistance from outside communities even though it does not address the need to reduce future vulnerability (McEntire et al. 2002). Indeed, cultural differences may be foundational in explaining the success or failure of a community in recovering from disaster (Jurkiewicz 2007; Kiefer and Montjoy 2006). Does this mean, simply, that richer communities will always bounce back faster and better?

I empathized—and still do empathize—with the City of New Orleans because I can so easily see something similar happening in Hampton Roads. After years of hurricane warnings and varying levels of outcomes, from mild (with great hurricane parties) to sobering (the flooding damage from Hurricane Isabel in 2003), suddenly the Big One arrives. Long-rehearsed plans are rolled into action. But there will always be some mundane, unexpected twist—the gasoline shortage, the incomplete road construction project that has road lanes blocked or otherwise unusable, the wicked storm surge that coincides disastrously with high tide—that escalates a really bad storm into something even worse, something horribly different, something exponentially more serious than anticipated. Does this mean we blame the victims? Do we see them as less deserving of empathy because they somehow brought the disaster on themselves, because they waited too long to evacuate, watching a capricious weather system as if they willed the hurricane onshore? Does this mean we force preparedness on individuals, driving buses into neighborhoods two days before the storm's anticipated landing and marching people from their homes with one carry-on bag apiece, no pets allowed?

In a way, this is the chorus of blame that fell on the heads and shoulders of New Orleanians. It was the "most predicted" disaster in American history (Cigler 2007, 64). They *knew* they were below sea level; they *knew* they were "sitting ducks" for a Category 4 or 5 hurricane; they *knew* their infrastructure, especially the levees, was in less-than-satisfactory condition. But, to paraphrase Jimmy Buffett, how do you reason with the hurricane season?

Barn Raising and Other Reciprocal Acts of Kindness

Americans are famously known for their independence and individualism. But, as the poet John Donne noted centuries ago, no man (*sic*) is an island, and sometimes we forget that America also has a strong tradition of community and what Daniel Kemmis (1990) called "barn raising," beautifully and even lovingly portrayed in the 1985 film *Witness*. In the film, the entire community comes together to build a barn for one family. Everyone helps, whether in the actual building of the barn or in cooking for and feeding the workers or minding the children. It is hot, hard work, but it is a social event, too. Everyone is willing, as each family has either benefited in the past, or knows it will benefit in the future, from similar acts of kindness from the community.

Eventually, even the most self-reliant among us reach a point when we can't go it alone. Sometimes, we need to ask for, and accept, help. Cheryl scolded me for my reluctance to accept help after my surgery and scolded me again when I admitted I would never have let a friend or child recover on his or her own. Social psychologists are not exactly sure how the acceptance of help translates into empathy, but they believe it typically begins at a very young age as mirroring behavior—a child mirrors the actions of his or her parent or other caregiver. At two to three years of age, a child can differentiate another's pain from his or her own and show signs of wanting to comfort the other. Children's empathetic responses are also affected by the responses of those around them; by imitating others, a child develops a repertoire of empathetic responses (Goleman 1997).

In mature individuals there is a distinction between cognitive and affective empathy. Cognitive empathy involves perspective taking ("I know what the other is feeling") and is more dispassionate; affective empathy ("I feel your pain") risks slipping into emotional contagion and personal distress. Other-oriented emotion has at times also been called "sympathy," "pity," and "compassion," but these don't have quite the same feel as empathy. There is also a distinction between acting out of empathy for another and acting to bolster one's own ego through the act of giving or helping.

What I particularly like about empathy is its root in mirroring behavior, and this is where I see it so compellingly connected to our national history and behavioral ethos. For all our rugged individualism, we could not conquer this continent and bring forth its promise as individuals. We had to bond together over a give-and-take of kindnesses, whether about clearing land, weaving cloth and quilting blankets, digging wells, or raising barns. I don't suggest that these mutual acts of kindness have disappeared—indeed, it is frequently in disaster situations that we see neighbors and strangers working together with chain saws to cut up fallen trees, fill sandbags and place them along the riverbank as the river rises toward flood stage, ferry others to safety in a boat after the flood crests, or slog through standing water to knock on doors to see who might be stranded and in need of help. It is in these moments that egoistic individualism falls away and the spirit of empathy we've cultivated comes shining through.

Public Administration

So, finally, what does the previous discussion have to do with public administration? I believe the answer is in one key word: mirroring.

Citizens in the contemporary age may speak the language of smaller government, but they expect a compassionate response from their public servants should they ever find themselves in need (King, Stivers, et al. 1998). The affiliated (if often unstated) question is, of course, whether citizens are willing to have their government spend taxpayer money to help *other* citizens in trouble, and if so, which citizens do they think deserve this help?

The answer, of course, is that *all* citizens deserve this help. When we look at many of the accepted roles of public administrators and public policy makers and the associated values, we typically see suggestions for responsibility, efficiency, accountability, discretion, and expertise. Yet the American Society for Public Administration's Code of Ethics calls for public servants to exercise compassion, benevolence, fairness, and optimism, and to consider future generations. These traits all call for empathy.

84   LISA A. ZANETTI

Training in disaster preparedness, for example, should include educating the broad teams of emergency managers, first responders, hazmat teams, public health officials—along with the expected mental health providers—about the importance of empathy and its appropriate boundaries. Media reports from disasters often include statements from survivors about how important it was for them to connect with someone who listened and cared about their ordeal.

Public service is a public trust. If we see public administrators as trustees of the public interest or ethical citizen-administrators charged with using moral imagination, then undoubtedly empathy is a foundational value. A discourse of care is not incompatible with the overall context of American history and political culture. We seldom see outright calls for empathy as a working value—yet arguably it is empathy that provides the foundation for altruism, tolerance, benevolence, and, by extension, public service.

Going back to the findings in neuroscience that empathy for those we perceive to be unlike ourselves is difficult to conjure, it seems to me there is a need—even an obligation—to cultivate that empathy, lest we relapse into a nation content to allow its inequities and inequalities to remain untouched. Problems also arise when empathy is not an openly articulated value, as this might allow hidden agendas and unequal treatment to persist. As an openly articulated value, however, a politics of empathy ensures that out-group members are viewed as sympathetically as in-group ones. Effectively, the part of the brain that censors affiliation with those perceived as different is consciously overridden.

Seventy years ago, the Italian theorist and political activist Antonio Gramsci noted that the law was at the intersection of the state and civil society, possessing the simultaneous potential for both coercion and transformation. In the current age, as government permeates nearly every aspect of life, Gramsci's observation might well be modified: it is public administration that is at the nexus of state and civil society. Public servants function as the mediators, in many instances, between the citizens and their elected representatives—and the reverse. They are in a unique position to perpetuate the status quo, or maneuver toward change. They can be the active sustainers of empathy as a normative value in public administration.

References

Ackerman, Diane. 2004. *An Alchemy of Mind: The Marvel and Mystery of the Brain.* New York: Scribner.

Batson, C.D., J. Chang, R. Orr, and J. Rowland. 2002. "Empathy, Attitudes and Action: Can Feeling for a Member of a Stigmatized Group Motivate One to Help the Group?" *Personality and Social Psychology Bulletin* 28 (12): 1656–66.

Cigler, Beverly. 2007. 'The "Big Questions' of Katrina and the 2005 Great Flood of New Orleans." *Public Administration Review* 67 (December): 64–76.

Geis, D. 2000. "By Design: The Disaster-Resistant and Quality-of-Life Community." *Natural Hazards Review* 1 (3): 151–60.

Gilligan, Carol. (1982) 1993. *In a Different Voice: Psychological Theory and Women's Development.* Cambridge, MA: Harvard University Press.

Goleman, Daniel. (1995) 1997. *Emotional Intelligence.* New York: Bantam Books.

Gutsell, Jennifer N., and Michael Inzlicht. 2010. "Empathy Constrained: Prejudice Predicts Reduced Mental Simulation of Actions during Observation of Outgroups." *Journal of Experimental Social Psychology* 46 (5): 841–45.

Hoffman, Martin L. 2000. *Empathy and Moral Development: Implications for Caring and Justice.* Cambridge, UK: Cambridge University Press.

Jurkiewicz, Carole. 2007. "Louisiana's Ethical Culture and Its Effect on the Administrative Failures Following Katrina." *Public Administration Review* 67 (December): 57–63.

Kemmis, Daniel. 1990. *Community and the Politics of Place.* Norman: University of Oklahoma Press.

Kiefer, J., and R. Montjoy. 2007. "Incrementalism before the Storm: Network Performance for the Evacuation of New Orleans." *Public Administration Review* 67 (December): 122–30.

King, Cheryl Simrell, Camilla Stivers, and Collaborators. 1998. *Government Is Us: Public Administration in an Anti-Government Era.* Thousand Oaks, CA: Sage.

Kristof, Nicholas. 2010. "A Scare, a Scar, a Silver Lining." *New York Times,* June 5. Available at http://www.nytimes.com/2010/06/06/opinion/06kristof.html, accessed July 23, 2010.

McEntire, D., C. Fuller, C. Johnston, and R. Weber. 2002. "A Comparison of Disaster Paradigms: The Search for a Holistic Policy Guide." *Public Administration Review* 2 (3): 267–81.

Noddings, Nel. 2002. *Educating Moral People.* New York: Teachers College Press.

Obama, Barack. 2008. *The Audacity of Hope: Thoughts on Reclaiming the American Dream.* New York: Vintage.

Pink, Daniel. 2006. *A Whole New Mind.* New York: Riverhead Trade.

Wolff, Janet. 1995. *Resident Alien: Feminist Cultural Criticism.* New Haven: Yale University Press.

6

Models of Citizen Participation

Measuring Engagement and Collaboration

Mary M. Timney

In the original *Government Is Us,* I described three models of citizen participation that I had uncovered while doing research on energy policy in the 1980s (Timney 1998). Since then, I have expanded the three—passive → hybrid → active—to a graduated scorecard. This model rates different methods of citizen participation that can be used to judge the level of involvement of citizens in a public process and the extent to which they are genuinely part of the decision-making process.

This chapter describes how the original models have been updated to a scorecard of participation on a scale of 0 to 10, from passive (0) to active (10). Two additional forms of citizen engagement are reviewed—the AmericaSpeaks method and the effective community governance model developed by Paul Epstein, Paul M. Coates, and Lyle D. Wray (2006). The scorecard is used to demonstrate how to evaluate different cases of citizen participation. This chapter concludes with a discussion of how administrators can use the scorecard to decide what kind of citizen engagement would be optimum in a given public decision-making situation.

Public Administration and Citizen Participation

From its earliest days, public administration established administrators as the experts in government or public policy implementation. The primary emphasis in the field has been the search for "the one best way" to do public management, whether in supervising employees, making optimal decisions, or designing programs or regulations in response to legislative mandates. Since the establishment of independent regulatory commissions in the late nineteenth century, the public administrator has been identified as the primary expert in the political arena: the cool-headed nonpartisan who can make the right decisions using professional criteria untainted by political pressures or ideology.

Guided by the dominant value in the field—efficiency—administrators developed processes for public review of agency proposals and decisions that achieve both the nominal requirements of democratic deliberation and the administrator's desire for efficiency. Increasingly today, lobbyists for corporate interests and contractors have much more influence over the development and implementation of public policy than ordinary citizens. Citizen participation is more prominent today but may be no more effective than in the past.

What Do We Mean By Citizen Participation?

The literature defines citizen participation in several ways, from the simple act of voting; to lobbying to affect political decisions; to actual involvement in decision making, as in a town meeting. Here the term *citizen participation* does not encompass lobbying but refers primarily to efforts to influence administrative decisions of policy-implementing agencies. Ned Crosby and colleagues (1986) distinguished the two. "Lobbying efforts are attempts to change public policy by getting large numbers of people to contact the appropriate public officials. The assumption is that a particular view is correct and the aim is to get as many supporters as possible to express this view to the public officials. Citizen participation . . . is an attempt to do the reverse: to start with a diverse group of people, inform them on the topic, and then get them to recommend that policy option which they find most appropriate" (Crosby, Kelly, and Schaefer 1986, 171). Lobbyists are generally paid to represent an interest while citizen participation is most often a volunteer activity. But even this definition no longer holds. Lobbyists can now organize "citizen groups" to storm representatives' offices and town meetings to protest pending legislation. This is called Astroturf roots to distinguish it from genuine grassroots political activity.

For most citizens, the reality of the public participation process rarely meets the promise of democracy. Public input in administrative decisions is likely to be solicited only after administrators and selected consultants have defined the problem and developed proposed solutions. Public participation is little more than a formality in many cases, designed to allow the public to comment while protecting the agency's interests. While citizens are given the opportunity to provide input, their suggestions rarely change the outcome of the process because the most critical decisions have usually been made already. As Daniel Kemmis, former mayor of Missoula, Montana, has observed, "Not much public listening goes on at the typical public hearing" (Stivers 1994, 368).

88   MARY M. TIMNEY

In a widely cited article, Sherry Arnstein (1969) described a ladder of citizen participation (see Figure 6.1). In her somewhat cynical observation, the lowest end of the scale is manipulation of public information, followed by therapy, informing, consultation, placation, partnership, and delegated power. Actual citizen control resides at the top of the ladder. Public managers rarely relinquish the control necessary to permit citizens to reach the top; until recently, even partnership has not been very common. Arnstein's ladder has become an icon in the fields of planning and public administration but has not been updated to account for new methods of citizen participation.

Models of Citizen Participation: Case Studies of State Energy Policy Development

In a 1992 study of state energy policy development, I found three distinct examples of citizen participation that formed a continuum from traditional agency-controlled citizen participation, to agency partnership with citizens in the advisory role, to citizen responsibility for policy development with the agency taking an advisory role. The three states from which the models were drawn were Ohio, Indiana, and Missouri.

Each state had similar goals for articulating state energy policy during a period free of federally mandated energy policy. Although their politics and energy vulnerability are different, the aim in each state was to develop a plan to integrate energy policy with environmental protection and economic development. Each used a different form of citizen participation with predictably different outcomes.

In Ohio, the governor appointed nine department secretaries to an ad hoc committee that met for eighteen months to develop the state energy strategy. During the closed administrative meetings, the committee consulted with other experts, principally representatives of the energy industries and large energy users. Politically, the state can be described as favoring economic development over environmental protection, and it is a major producer and exporter of electricity. The aim of the energy strategy process was to protect state business interests while developing ideas for complying with new environmental protection laws.

Two rounds of public hearings were held across the state. The committee made the final recommendations and developed a policy document that favored industry interests and emphasized economic development. The citizens' comments were included in an appendix to the report. Few, if any, changes were made in the final proposal as a result of the public input.

The state of Indiana is similar to Ohio in energy resources and politics. The state's utilities export electricity, and the state is a major coal producer. Thus

MODELS OF CITIZEN PARTICIPATION   89

Figure 6.1   **Components of Arnstein's Ladder of Participation**

Citizen Power

 8 Citizen Control

 7 Delegated Power

Tokenism

 5 Placation

 4 Consultation

Nonparticipation

 2 Therapy

 1 Manipulation

Source: Adapted from Arnstein 1969.

the incentives to develop an energy policy were very much the same as those in Ohio. However, in Indiana, the process was initiated by the chair of the state senate who wanted to develop a consensual decision process for contentious policy issues. Energy was not a politically hot issue at the time, although energy industries have considerable power in the Indiana legislature.

In this case, however, the focus was as much on the process itself as on the policy. The energy agency, which is housed in the department of commerce, was charged with designing a way to maximize citizen participation. The agency identified relevant publics to be involved, drafted discussion documents, and set up task forces to develop recommendations for the state

90   MARY M. TIMNEY

energy policy. Membership on the task forces was open to anyone willing to participate. Ultimately, more than 200 people from all economic and social sectors worked on the final product. The agency's decisions were greatly informed by the consensus reports of the task forces. Both the director of the Hoosier Environmental Council and the chief lobbyist for the electricity industry told me how well the process worked to help them to understand each other's viewpoint.

The case of Missouri represents the other extreme of the continuum from controlled to open participation and citizen decision making. Following normal procedure, the department of energy administrators drafted working materials that defined the problems, proposed alternatives, and generally limited the parameters of the discussion—just what managers are trained and expected to do. At this point, however, they departed from tradition: they contracted out the citizen participation element of the process to a citizens' organization, the Kansas City Metropolitan Energy Center (MEC). The MEC identified a set of relevant publics across the state—business, labor, environmental groups, chambers of commerce, small businesses, and so forth—much the way an administrator would do. But the similarities ended there. These individuals were then asked to identify who *they* thought should be involved in the process.

A series of more than thirty focus groups was held throughout the state to review the administrators' recommendations and develop consensus on implementation options. At first, many of the participants felt that the discussion papers were a draft of the final report that they were being asked to approve or modify. However, MEC personnel structured the meetings to develop comments and inputs from the participants; facilitators of the discussions focused on *listening, rather than presenting,* information.

In the end, the focus groups rejected the priorities of the agency administrators, restructured the study outline, and redirected the presentation of the materials. Citizen participation was so powerful in this case that the seven-volume final report was then written by the MEC, not the state energy agency. And because this was a consensual process that developed political support across the state, the legislature quickly enacted most of the recommendations (State of Missouri Department of Natural Resources 1992). In this case, citizen participation occurred at the top rung of Arnstein's (1969) ladder.

From these cases, I developed a set of citizen participation models to describe what happened. Table 6.1 shows the characteristics of each level, dividing them along a continuum from passive to active. At the time, I named the Indiana case the hybrid or transition model. Today, I see it as an example of the collaborative network paradigm, which is described in the scorecard presented later. The important descriptor in this model is that Indiana represents government *with* the people.

Table 6.1

Characteristics of Citizen Participation Models

Active	Hybrid (transition)	Passive
Missouri	Indiana	Ohio
• Citizen control	• Shared control	• Agency control
• Citizens identify parameters	• Agency identifies parameters	• Agency identifies parameters
• Proactive, open	• Broad, open process	• Closed process
• Consensus decisions	• Consensus decisions	• Access limited
• Citizen role is dominant	• Citizen role advisory	• Citizens react to proposals
• Agency serves as consultant	• Administrators articulate policy	• Administrators articulate policy
• Citizens articulate policy	• Administrators as staff and participants	• Expert decisions
• Citizens own the process	• Expert decisions informed by the public	• Participation as formality
• Citizens come in at beginning of process	• Participation as process goal	• Citizens come at end of process
	• Citizens come in middle of process	
Government by the people	Government with the people	Government for the people

Source: Timney 1998.

A quick scan of these states' Web sites reveals that not much has changed in fifteen years. The Ohio Energy Office has a link on the Web page to energy efficiency, and Indiana's Office of Energy Development appears to still be focused on increasing business opportunities. Missouri has the Energy Policy Office, a nonprofit organization, under the Department of Natural Resources that has links to a range of energy-efficiency and alternative-energy programs. There are several boards and commissions in Missouri that involve citizens at the highest policy levels. It appears that once you let citizens in the door, they're going to stay.

Expanding the Models

When I moved to the New York metropolitan area in 2002, I became involved with the Civic Alliance, a citizens' organization in Lower Manhattan that was working to involve citizens in decision making for the rebuilding of the World Trade Center site. They were developing scorecards for various stages of the rebuilding effort, and they asked me to draft one for citizen participation. They wanted to be able to track the progress of different phases of the

92   MARY M. TIMNEY

reconstruction to measure how much public input was being adopted in the rebuilding effort.

They had just been through an empowering process with America*Speaks* called "Listening to the City" in the summer of 2002. This process involved 5,000 citizens meeting over a day and a half, sitting around small tables connected by computers. The process produced consensus on several ideas that were then reviewed by the Lower Manhattan Development Corporation (LMDC), an agency appointed by former Governor George Pataki to lead the rebuilding effort.

The citizens were anxious to keep the involvement momentum going. A group of us brainstormed about different types of citizen participation. Some, such as e-voting for different building designs, were being used by LMDC. We discussed how to get all "citizens" involved in the discussion, especially residents of Chinatown, who are often overlooked, and immigrants for whom English is a second language. In our view, all residents were considered to be citizens, legal or not. We began to refer to public participation as a way to get around the designation of citizens as legal entities. As a result of this collaboration, I developed the Scorecard of Citizen Participation Methods (Table 6.2).

The scorecard runs from 0 to 10. The first three scores represent total agency control of the process. The scorecard begins with noncommunicating at Level 0. At Level 1, informing reflects noninteractive reporting by agencies. Level 2 provides one-way feedback, typical of an agency receiving comments to a rulemaking published in the Federal Register. Segmented consultation occurs at Level 3 and usually involves experts, business groups, and, increasingly, corporate lobbyists. Organized citizen groups may be included to keep the process legitimate.

Levels 4 through 7 demonstrate an increasing level of citizen engagement but there is still very little conversation or collaboration at this stage. Formal procedures on Level 4 represent traditional public hearings. Level 5 describes feedback through the media in which public comment is solicited by agencies or other entities (talk shows, electronic petitions, e-voting, etc.). These are unscientific and often represent extreme positions, and some are manipulated by the media. Scientific feedback is placed at Level 6 where agencies use surveys of randomly selected participants. This would not include the type of so-called push polling used by elected representatives with their constituents to gain support for their positions. Finally, Level 7 is used for interactive processes in which selected citizens are chosen to participate in focus groups or other group exercises to provide feedback to the agency. This doesn't rise to the level of collaboration because it is still controlled by the agency, which makes the ultimate decisions; the agency is perhaps better informed by the process. These levels generally follow the model of managerial decision

Table 6.2 Scorecard of Citizen Participation Methods

	Type of method	Description	Characteristics
Active			
10	Delegated power	Public decision making	Agency[a] delegates decision making to public groups through contracting; partici-pants selected by the public; open processes; agency delegates decision power
Collaborative Network Paradigm (8–9)			
9	Collaboration	Public/agency decision making	Iterative processes in which public and agency learn through feedback and arrive at a consensus; participants selected by both public and agency; open processes; agency shares decision power
8	Partnership (advisory)	Agency decision making informed by public through organized processes	Advisory working groups meeting in structured events; participants selected by both public and agency; open processes; agency retains decision power, but is strongly influenced by the products of the process
Passive			
Unitary or Inclusive Consultation (4–7)			
7	Interactive	Agency solicits public input through structured process	Focus groups; participants selected by agency but may be solicited openly; agency retains decision power and may or may not be influenced by input
6	Scientific feedback	Agency solicits public input through social science methods	Scientific surveys designed to identify broad public concerns; participants ran-domly selected
5	Feedback through media	Opportunities for public comment not controlled by agency	Talk shows; unscientific media surveys; Web-based threaded discussions; e-voting; participants self-selected
4	Formal procedures	Agency solicits public input in an open meeting	Public hearings; participants self-selected
3	Segmented consultation	Agency solicits input from experts and/or representatives of selected interest groups	Expert advisory groups; corporate lobbyists; agency selects individuals or groups for consultation; agency makes decision and may be influenced by participants
2	One-way feedback	Agency solicits feedback to identify preferences	Informal voting processes; written comments; unshared responses to Web sites; participants self-selected; agency makes decision, may or may not be influenced
1	Informing	Agency provides information to public about decisions	Reports; public meetings; Web site (noninteractive); decision has already been made by agency
0	Noncom-municating	Closed process	Unilateral decision; no advance public information

[a]Agency refers to any formal entity, public or private.

94   MARY M. TIMNEY

making outlined by John Clayton Thomas (1995) in *Public Participation in Public Decisions.* The passive section of the scorecard thus ranges from 0 to 7, principally because the agency controls the processes and there is no actual collaboration with citizens.

The active section of the scorecard begins at Level 8. This level (partnership) and Level 9 (collaboration) are designated as the collaborative network paradigm (CNP); the hybrid case of the original models belongs at Level 8. The CNP represents interaction between agency and citizens, where all participants are considered to be equal members of the discourse—businessmen and environmentalists, rich women and social workers, gardeners and cleaning women. Each is considered to hold valuable pieces of public information to inform and improve decisions.

These could be the kinds of listening sessions described by John Forester (1999) in *The Deliberative Practitioner,* in which he tries to educate his planning students about learning to understand the richness of the lived experience. Forester collected cases of planning around the world and presents them as examples of what happens when planners listen to the indigenous people rather than their leaders.

At base, then, the CNP requires that there be space for citizens to come together and the time to give all participants the opportunity to contribute to the discourse. This should not be a Habermasian discourse where the best idea wins the day (see Habermas 1998); rather, it derives more from the philosophy of James Bohman (1996), who argues for the design of a "discursive public space" in which everyone affected by a decision has "equal opportunities to participate in deliberation, equality in methods of decision making and in determining the agenda, the free and open exchange of information and reasons sufficient to acquire an understanding of both the issue in question and the opinions of others" (16).

Level 9 (collaboration) requires a process that is iterative, occurs over time, and allows the agency and citizens to learn together as the discourse progresses. It is open, with participants having many opportunities to come into the deliberation. Its decision making is ongoing as projects are implemented and conditions change. Most importantly, the decision making is so consensual that it is impossible in the final outcome to determine which part came from the citizens or any segment of the public and which from the agency. It is the type of consensus described by Mary Parker Follett (1926) in *The New State.* Follett argues that compromise outcomes represent the combination of what neither side wants; each participant has to give up something it may really want to reach a compromise. All leave the table feeling worse off. Consensus, on the other hand, occurs when all participants seek an outcome that is greater than the sum of the parts, a synergistic result that leaves everyone better off. Contemporary negotiators call this win–win negotiation (Fisher, Ury, and Patton 1991).

Level 9 (collaboration) is likely to be expensive and time-consuming the first time it is tried. After one successful effort, however, participants are likely to want to work together on other problems and the learning curve will not be as steep for the later processes. When citizens begin to trust administrators and administrators learn to listen to citizens, developing and implementing public policy becomes easier, more efficient, and more effective. It is always much more expensive and time-consuming to try to implement a project that is contentious, especially if it turns into a NIMBY situation.

Level 10 (delegated power) describes the active case in the earlier model. Here the agency turns over the decision to the citizens and serves in an advisory role. The agency then implements the decision. In 1995, I saw this as the ideal—government *by* the people. I now believe that collaboration is the ideal—government *with* the people. This collaboration may help to escape from the political perception that government bureaucrats are somehow the enemy. It also recognizes that government administrators are also citizens and that their expertise has value in the decision-making process.

The *America*Speaks *Method*

To illustrate the use of the scorecard, we now examine two approaches to citizen participation: the America*Speaks* method and the effective community governance model. America*Speaks* (www.americaspeaks.org) is a nonprofit organization whose mission is "reinvigorating American democracy by engaging citizens in the public decisions that most impact their lives." Their approach is to set up large-scale meetings, called 21st Century Town Meetings.

These meetings are designed to involve up to several thousand people broken into groups of ten to twelve participants. Each group has a facilitator and an electronic link to a central processor. The participants engage in face-to-face discussions of issues from public policy, to budgeting to planning, and so on. The results are quickly summarized and reported to all participants and government representatives, elected and professional, who are present. Citizens have meaningful input into government decisions that impact their lives. Two examples of these meetings were Listening to the City in New York in the summer of 2002 and the Washington DC Citizen Summits on the city budget.

Washington, DC Citizen Summits

"In 1999, Washington, D.C. Mayor Anthony Williams launched a process to renew people's faith in government and to get them personally involved

96   MARY M. TIMNEY

in changing life in the District. In partnership with America*Speaks,* over the course of six years the Mayor's office held seven D.C.-wide 21st Century Town Meetings, through which more than 13,500 residents deliberated about the city's spending priorities and made recommendations for change" (America*Speaks* 2010). One of the meetings was designated for Washington youth. As a result of these summits, public input led to better budget allocations and the formation of new community-based governance mechanisms, such as the Office of Neighborhood Action.

Using the scorecard, we can place the DC Citizen Summits at Level 9. The meetings took place over several years with participants continuously learning how to build consensus. The citizen input changed the priorities of budget allocations and led to the creation of a new Office of Neighborhood Action. The process has continued annually without America*Speaks.*

Listening to the City

This project was developed to bring together community interests around the rebuilding of the World Trade Center site after September 11, 2001. The concern among citizens groups and professional planners at the time was that business and political interests would prevail over broader community interests, including those of the families of the victims who perished in the attacks. In the spring of 2002, the Lower Manhattan Development Corporation (LMDC) proposed six building designs that raised serious concerns among the public about the future of the site.

America*Speaks* convened three meetings. The first one involved 600 "community leaders, issue advocates and planning professionals" (America*Speaks* 2010). As a result of these meetings, which demonstrated the value of citizen input, LMDC and the Port Authority, the owner of the World Trade Center site, cosponsored a second meeting as a central feature of the citizen engagement process. This meeting involved 4,500 members of the general public who closely reflected the demographic diversity of the region and provided input on site plans. This was followed by a two-week online dialogue that reached "another 800 New York City residents who reviewed the site options in small cybergroups" (America*Speaks* 2010).

The results showed that the "participants of Listening to the City demonstrated the public's desire for more vision and imagination than the six different proposed plans offered." Among the principles shaped by the people were "preserving the footprints of the Twin Towers for memorial-related space, restoring a powerful, tall symbol in Lower Manhattan's skyline and reestablishing the street grid and improving connectivity within Lower Manhattan" (America*Speaks* 2010).

None of the six proposed plans incorporated all of these elements so LMDC launched an Innovative Design Study. The final design by Daniel Libeskind incorporated these elements and others of those articulated by the public at Listening to the City. The town meeting was hailed at the time as a model for the future and an innovative way to build consensus among large groups that had never seemed possible before.

The Citizens Alliance, formed in Lower Manhattan by the Regional Plan Association (www.rpa.org), hoped to carry this momentum forward through ongoing involvement in the decision process. In the spring and summer of 2004, LMDC (www.renewnyc.com) held a series of smaller meetings on its own that involved interested citizens in different neighborhoods throughout Lower Manhattan. These meetings, with facilitators, focused on the mix of commercial, cultural, and residential uses that citizens wanted to see in the neighborhood of the site.

Listening to the City is harder to place on the scale in relation to the collaborative network paradigm. It appears to be closer to Level 8 since it does not seem that administrators were involved in the process, so the outcomes were advisory. It is true that the response from LMDC, the Port Authority, and the governor was to adopt many of the principles in the redesign of the site, but there is no evidence that the citizens were engaged in an ongoing process with decision makers. The later meetings and other participation efforts (there was a Level 5 electronic vote for the final designs) were advisory. The 2004 meetings were closer to Level 7 (focus groups) than collaborative.

Effective Community Governance Model

This model was developed by Paul Epstein, Paul M. Coates, and Lyle D. Wray (2006) to describe the interactions among organizations, citizens, and professionals in community problem solving with measurable results. Their book, *Results that Matter: Improving Communities by Engaging Citizens, Measuring Performance, and Getting Things Done,* presents a set of real-world cases and uses the model to demonstrate how communities have engaged citizens in creating meaningful lasting change on issues identified as important to and by the citizens.

The model, shown in Figure 6.2, is a Venn diagram with three concentric circles that represent core community skills: engaging citizens, measuring results, and getting things done by both the private and public sectors.

Advanced governance practices occur at the overlaps of the circles. Level 1 (community problem solving) occurs at the overlap of engaging citizens and getting things done. Citizens play an influential role in what gets done but they may have to advocate to policy makers for implementation. There

Figure 6.2 **Effective Community Governance Model**

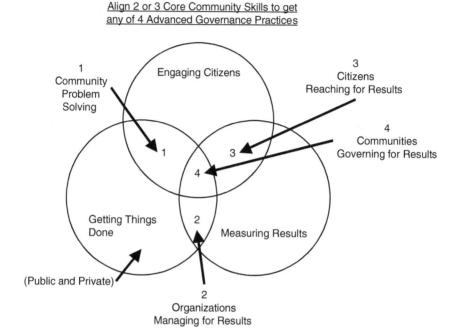

Source: Epstein et al. 2006.

may be no results measurement and thus no performance feedback into community decision making (Epstein et al. 2006, 7).

Level 2, organizations managing for results, comes at the alignment of the getting things done and measuring results circles. Citizens are primarily engaged as stakeholders but results measurement provides data on community outcomes and program performance. Feedback can show where collaboration is needed but it is primarily a tool for organizational improvement. "While this practice can be very effective at achieving measurable results, results achieved do not necessarily reflect citizens' main concerns, because citizens are not involved in framing issues or setting priorities" (Epstein et al. 2006, 8).

Level 3 (citizens reaching for results) is where citizens decide what results get measured, collect results data, decide what data to use for advocacy, or use the data themselves to build collaborations with other groups. Since measures are not systematically connected to organizations or resources to achieve desired results, citizen engagement occurs as advocacy (Epstein et al. 2006, 8).

At Level 4 (communities governing for results), at the intersection of all three circles, the desired outcome is created by aligning citizens who are engaged in identifying what gets measured and who sometimes participate in measuring results and ongoing collaborations with the organization(s) implementing the policies. "Collaborations tend to be results focused and are likely to include both collaborations among organizations and between citizens and organizations" (Epstein et al. 2006, 9).

Organizations and cases highlighted in Epstein's work include, among others, the Jacksonville Community Council Inc. (Level 1); the San Jose Department of Streets and Traffic (Epstein et al. 2006, 49) (Level 2); the Iowa Citizen-Initiated Performance Assessment project (Level 3); and the Prince William County, Virginia, Governing for Results Cycles (Epstein et al. 2006, 140ff) (Level 4).

Each of these levels can be placed on the scorecard. Only Epstein's Practice 4, Communities Governing for Results, falls comfortably in the collaborative network paradigm, ideally at Level 9 on the scorecard, where citizens are actively engaged with administrators, public and private, in all stages of policy decisions. Two other practices described by Epstein, community problem solving and citizens reaching for results, involve advocacy, which is not represented on the scorecard. Advocacy can't be placed in Level 10 since it is not delegated power per se. At the same time, advocacy groups that produce studies or proposals that are ultimately used by the local government for community improvement are collaborating and engaged. Epstein's Practice 2, organizations managing for results, occurs at the lower levels of the scorecard (Levels 1, 2 and/or 3). Agencies (public and private) may provide feedback to the community or solicit input from citizens, but this part of the model does not involve significant citizen engagement.

The community governance model and the cases described by Epstein and colleagues provide guidance to citizens' groups and organizations committed to engaging citizens in robust processes to improve their communities.

Using the Scorecard to Evaluate Citizen Participation

The scorecard provides a tool for administrators and citizen organizations that are truly committed to collaborative decision making. Every decision of government does not require a collaborative process, but projects or plans that are likely to have significant effects on citizens probably require more discussion than provided by a typical administrative hearing (Level 4).

Administrators can use the scorecard to evaluate the ways that they involve citizens in projects that affect their communities: Are all citizen input sessions controlled and managed by time or format? How are citizens' opinions weighed in decision making? Has the community had NIMBY problems in the past? Why have they occurred? How could collaborative processes have ameliorated these situations? The scorecard levels can help administrators to design the type of participation that would be most desirable in a given situation.

Citizen organizations can use the scorecard to identify the type of process that they might want to advocate for in specific cases. If citizens find that they are continually on the outside trying to be heard, it may be worthwhile to meet with administrators or political leaders to discuss the scorecard levels. Getting the support of other groups to advocate for a higher level of citizen participation might also be effective in persuading government leaders to work more collaboratively with citizens. The scorecard gives citizens a tool with which to identify the kind of participation that would be most worthy of their efforts. One of the reasons that citizens don't get involved more is the conviction that their input is not valued. Working to create better methods will help to get more citizens involved in the future of their communities.

References

America*Speaks*. 2010. http://www.americaspeaks.org/index.cfm?fuseaction=Page. viewPage&pageId=499&parentID=473&nodeID=1 (accessed June 30, 2010).

Arnstein, Sherry R. 1969. "A Ladder of Citizen Participation." *Journal of the American Institute of Planners* 35 (4): 216–24.

Bohman, James. 1996. *Public Deliberation: Pluralism, Complexity, and Democracy.* Cambridge, MA: The MIT Press.

Crosby, Ned, J.M. Kelly, and P. Schaefer. 1986. "Citizen Panels: A New Approach to Citizen Participation." *Public Administration Review* 46 (2): 170–78.

Epstein, Paul D., Paul M. Coates, and Lyle D. Wray. 2006. *Results that Matter: Improving Communities by Engaging Citizens, Measuring Performance, and Getting Things Done.* San Francisco: Jossey-Bass.

Fisher, R., William Ury, and B. Patton. 1991. *Getting to Yes: Negotiating Agreement without Giving In.* 2d ed. New York: Penguin Books.

Follett, Mary Parker. 1926. *The New State: Group Organization; the Solution of Popular Government.* 5th ed. New York: Longmans, Green.

Forester, John. 1999. *The Deliberative Practitioner: Encouraging Participatory Planning Processes.* Cambridge, MA: The MIT Press.

Habermas, Jurgen. 1998. *Between Facts and Norms: Contributions to a Discourse Theory of Law and Democracy,* trans. William Rehg. Cambridge, MA: The MIT Press.

State of Missouri Department of Natural Resources. 1992. "Public Participation." In *Missouri Statewide Energy Study,* vol. 6. Jefferson City, MO: Environmental Improvement and Energy Resources Authority.

Stivers, Camilla. 1994. "The Listening Bureaucrat: Responsiveness in Public Administration." *Public Administration Review* 54: 364–69.

Thomas, John Clayton. 1995. *Public Participation in Public Decisions.* San Francisco: Jossey-Bass.

Timney, Mary. 1998. "Overcoming Administrative Barriers to Citizen Participation: Citizens as Partners, Not Adversaries." In *Government Is Us: Public Administration in an Anti-government Era,* ed. Cheryl Simrell King, Camilla Stivers, and Collaborators. Thousand Oaks, CA: Sage.

7

Democratic Governance through Public-Nonprofit Partnerships

Reclaiming "A Usable Past" from the Settlement House Movement

Jennifer K. Alexander

This case study presents a modern-day example of democratic governance practiced in the tradition of the settlement house movement and demonstrates how it revived a county human service agency that was in crisis. The story is drawn from findings of a ten-year longitudinal study of partnerships forged between a county agency and nine community-based nonprofits between 1998 and 2008. All partnerships were established with the same agency, county child welfare (CWA), for the same purpose, to provide community-based child welfare services.

Current literature elaborates the benefits of public-nonprofit partnerships from an instrument perspective; they are regarded as a short-term, less expensive means of delivering services. Contractual partnerships enable administrators to "steer rather than row" and to encourage market mechanisms to guide public programs. Largely occluded in the present literature is the more substantive contribution of public-nonprofit partnerships. They can provide an opportunity for democratic governance and resolve the challenge of governance failure, defined not in the context of a market model, but as the failure of the public sector to successfully establish relationships of trust and accountability. Accountability in this circumstance is defined as confidence on the part of citizens that government will act in their best interests or take action in accordance with shared values.

There is a wealth of literature that documents a lack of trust in government, most particularly where it is entrenched among traditional minority populations (Alexander 1997; Alexander and Nank 2009; King, Stivers, and Collaborators 1998). Administrative policies and procedures directed to those

102   JENNIFER K. ALEXANDER

not originally afforded the privileges of citizenship have a history of reliance on police power, and the present case of child welfare is a prototypical example. Child welfare agencies are regulatory human service agencies with an adversarial mission, most often engaged with marginalized populations, and agency-citizen relationships are characteristically involuntary and coercive, and pertain to intimate aspects of people's lives. The partnerships established in this case study provide a particularly fertile example of how a regulatory agency transitioned from control to a politics of engagement. The achievement of democratic governance in this circumstance fits what Flyvbjerg referred to as a "least likely" case for success (Flyvbjerg 2004, 26). If practices of democratic governance can flourish in these partnerships, the methods and lessons may be applicable to a variety of other organizational contexts that pertain to human services and marginalized populations.

This chapter provides a brief review of the core ideas that traverse the history of public administration, from the settlement house movement through the New Public Service. We investigate the practice of citizenship and how mediating institutions play a critical role as a nexus between the public sector and citizens, legitimating the lived experience of residents and fostering democratic knowledge. We also explore the responsibilities of public administrators and the idea that public administration is a practical endeavor intended to improve people's lives. I provide a background on the case study and how it was conducted. An unusual story illustrates a public-nonprofit partnership that recaptured the buried heritage of the settlement house movement and became a national model of success in child welfare.

During the Progressive era a group of urban reformers known as settlement workers sought to better the lives of lower-income residents by living with them and learning about their daily challenges firsthand. These early reformers sought to create a neighborhood spirit; a community engaged in mutual aid. Settlement workers believed that through this approach they could understand the conditions and causes of poverty and advocate for more effective policy (Stivers 2002). They took their work as a form of good citizenship; in fact, they regarded it as the central organizing point for public administration. While their ideas about the purpose and role of public administration were eventually overshadowed by the approach of the bureau men, the zeitgeist of the settlement house movement has reemerged in the literature as the New Public Service (NPS). NPS views public administration as a form of democratic governance; administrators are advised to engage citizens in the task of defining the ends of government with the intention of creating a better life for all (Denhardt and Denhardt 2007, 4).

Scholarship in the vein of New Public Service has advocated for active engagement of citizens in the task of governance (Cooper 1998; Stivers

2002). Administrators share authority with a citizenry and foster a sense of responsibility to their political community (King, Stivers, and Collaborators 1998; Box 1998; Frederickson and Chandler 1984). The New Public Service affirms the importance of mediating structures and community that provide a collective identity for citizens (Kantor 1972; Sandel 1981; Wolin 1994). These associations provide a setting within which citizens can articulate their concerns, solve problems, and transmit democratic knowledge to government where it informs policy. Much like the settlement house workers who preceded, advocates of democratic governance view administrators as public servants, citizens themselves who eschew the traditional forms of hierarchy and expertise in favor of horizontal relationships with citizens (Cooper 1998; Denhardt and Denhardt 2007). A final theme that wends through the writings of early settlement workers to present-day scholars who advocate for democratic governance is the commitment to a government that betters people's lives.

This chapter illuminates four less-developed aspects of democratic governance. It reveals a process by which connection between public administrators and citizens can be fostered, how mediating institutions support citizen administrator interactions in a manner that facilitates the open dialogue necessary to generate democratic knowledge, how the use of that knowledge has informed public agency decisions, and how the role of public administrators has changed.

Background

In 1998 a county child welfare agency (CWA) in a large midwestern city was selected by the Annie E. Casey Foundation to participate in a national pilot program intended to redesign child welfare services. The intention of the Family to Family (F2F) initiative was to shift child welfare services from an adversarial, problem-oriented approach with the intention of protecting children, to a community-based, prevention-oriented approach intended to build family and community capacity to raise children (DeMuro 1995). The Annie E. Casey Foundation encouraged public sector agencies in five states that were particularly burdened to pursue their mission through community building in partnership with mediating institutions. In this case, the logical partners were multiservice community centers, or community-based organizations (CBOs) with a tradition of serving their communities since their founding as settlement houses at the turn of the nineteenth century.

The F2F partnerships were exceptional for three reasons. First, the terms of the partnership were not defined or funded by government; a private foundation conceptualized the approach and provided resources for the initiative. Second, F2F established partnerships that were both substantive and con-

104   JENNIFER K. ALEXANDER

tractual in nature. Over the course of a decade, the public agency and CBOs progressively integrated task responsibilities and authority to institutionalize collaborative decision making. At the conclusion of the investigation in 2008, CBO staff members were serving on county agency policy-making boards and on hiring and promotion committees within the public agency, and CBO representatives were granted veto power on CWA mid- to senior-level agency appointments. Finally, the F2F partnerships in this particular county were sustained for the longest duration without interruption, which afforded the opportunity to identify long-term results.

The investigation of the F2F initiative began in 1998 when the CWA that is the subject of this study came under a barrage of criticism from local political figures, the media, and urban community leaders due to the deaths of several children who had open cases with the agency. One county commissioner denounced the public agency in the press and asserted that "children would be better off in orphanages," and that "social workers in the agency were morons" (American Humane Association 1998, 7). It was the daunting task before this particular agency that made for an intriguing study. How would an embattled CWA achieve its mission in partnership with mediating institutions that represented the interests of a community? Would public administration leaders be successful in their efforts to change the pattern of interaction within this agency from regulation and control over citizens to community engagement? We decided to track the progress of the public-nonprofit partnerships to understand how they were established, how they evolved, and their effect on the agency's capacity to fulfill its mission.

The midwestern county that is the subject of this study is among the fifteen largest county governments in the United States and encompasses one of the five poorest big cities. This city was ranked among the bottom five of fifty U.S. cities according to indicators of children's well-being (Annie E. Casey Foundation 1997). The county began two pilot F2F partnerships in 1998, and seven more followed between 1999 and 2004. By 2004, the need for a community-based model of child welfare had expanded into the suburban areas and the CWA sought new lead agency partners. Unfortunately, the suburbs lacked multiservice nonprofits with deep community roots and a history of providing a wide array of services for families. The executive director of the CWA encouraged suburban municipalities to identify likely mediating institutions, and four municipalities instituted new partnerships with the CWA; two school districts, a youth services division of a local government, and a police department partnered with a local YMCA.

The case study was developed from document reviews, participant observation that occurred at the CWA, the CBOs, community gatherings held to elaborate the initiative, and three phases of semi-structured interviews conducted between October 1998 and November 2008. In 1998, at the inception of the study, a series of interviews were conducted with the county agency staff, the F2F liaison within the county agency, and staff located at the first two CBO pilot partnerships. We maintained minimal contact with the partnership between 1999 and 2003 and then returned to conduct a second round of interviews in the spring of 2004 with the county leadership and staff, the first two pilot CBOs, and the seven new CBOs that had become partners of the CWA. The third phase of interviews began in the fall of 2007 and explored how differences between municipal and nonprofit lead agency shaped the partnerships. Three CBOs selected for this final round most typified all CBOs in the partnership with respect to (1) their interactions with the CWA; (2) range of services; and (3) the service population. In addition, interviews were conducted with three new municipal lead agencies that had joined the partnership in 2004. They included two school districts and a Division of Youth within the Human Services Department of a municipality.

Interviews were conducted in person and then prepared as written documents, which were then returned to interviewees to discern whether the researchers had accurately captured their perspectives and experience. In the following section I review how the public agency built a connection with the community, the role of the CBOs (formerly settlement houses) as institutions that mediated between the public agency and the community they represented, the generation of democratic knowledge that improved administrative decision making, and how democratic governance changed the roles of public administrators.

Bridging the Gap: Fostering a Connection with Citizens

Scholars in the tradition of democratic governance have argued that public administrators are in a vital position to foster active citizenship (Cooper 1991; Denhardt and Denhardt 2000; Frederickson 1997; King, Stivers, and Collaborators 1998; Stivers 2000). It is through the practice of citizenship that people develop a public identity and a capacity to discern the common good. Democratic governance rests on the premise that public administrators discern what to do based on information drawn from an ongoing and forthright dialogue with citizens. But how do administrators foster active citizenry, and how might this relationship with a community of citizens be established?

The intention of the F2F partnerships was to shift from a model where the care and protection of children rested with a public agency to one of shared responsibility with the community. The CWA needed to generate a neighborhood commitment to mutual aid and support for protecting children by building family and community capacity to nurture and care for them. The first challenge for the public agency, however, was to bridge the chasm of distrust between the public agency and the community by interesting community leaders, many of whom were CBO executive directors and ministers, in the idea of the partnership.

As we attended the community meetings at the beginning of the F2F initiative, the extent to which citizens and the African American community in particular distrusted the county agency was readily apparent. Executive directors of CBOs and other community members spoke of how county social workers were arbitrary, autocratic, and unwilling or unable to act in the best interests of families or children. Nobody, including social workers who worked for nonprofit agencies engaged in child welfare services, seemed to comprehend the logic behind CWA decisions regarding risk assessments or child custody. Moreover, there was marked disagreement as to the extent to which child abuse was a problem. One executive director of a CBO went so far as to state that the intention of the CWA was to take "black babies and give them to white people in the suburbs."

The executive director of the CWA, in a prescient moment, hired a well-known community advocate as the F2F liaison between the CWA and the community. The advocate, Theresa, was an African American woman and a licensed social worker who had established and directed a number of family-related programs over twenty years. In her capacity as internal coordinator, Theresa gave the community and mediating institutions a sense that they had an educated advocate inside the county agency. Theresa promoted the new F2F initiative in widely publicized meetings held in churches and community centers where she, in the company of local ministers and social workers, told an empowering story:

> This initiative is a means for us to build our community's strength to care for our children. Family to Family will help us build the strength of our community to nurture our children so that with time, the county's role will progressively shrink away.

What we found most compelling about Theresa's message was her unbroken affiliation with the community and her primary commitment to helping them build networks of mutual aid and support. She did not ask the citizens to trust the county, but to join together as a community to take control of the fate of their children.

Theresa built community capacity by creating "collaboratives," or networks of community residents, social service agencies, churches, businesses, and schools that provided services and programs at the CBOs. The collaboratives provided parenting classes, day care services and activities for children, and training for potential foster parents. They built awareness within neighborhood institutions about the challenges of their children. The collaboratives enhanced programs available through the CBO for families under stress and continuity for children who had been removed from their homes. For example, children who needed to be removed from their homes could be placed with a foster family and remain in their own neighborhood, maintaining critical ties with school, family, friends, and activities.

One of the more compelling examples of how F2F generated mutual aid within neighborhoods involved the relationships that were built between foster and biological families. In marked contrast to previous CWA policy, which prohibited contact or sharing information between biological and foster families, F2F encouraged relationships that supported the interest of the children. Foster parents, who were most often older couples in the neighborhood, mentored young mothers, provided coaching, and helped them learn parenting skills. When children were reunited with their biological parents, foster parents remained available to provide weekend respite care for the children, thus developing a neighborhood network of support for children and their parents.

Reviving a Public Service based on Community, Care, and Advocacy

In *Bureau Men, Settlement Women,* Stivers (2002) argued that early visions of the task and goals of government were heavily gendered. While bureau men viewed the work of public administration through the lens of business and industry, settlement house workers, who were primarily women, saw the city as a home. Bureau men approached public administration with the intention of generating an objective body of knowledge, a science of administration equipped with techniques and methods that would foster expertise and improve the efficiency and effectiveness of practice. Proper administration would issue from science, reason, expertise, and careful attention to the means rather than the ends of state action.

Settlement workers believed government was intended to improve the quality of human life. As the work of a home, settlement workers regarded public administration as a moral endeavor and sought a public conscience in service and programs. "Probation systems should be staffed by people who thought of themselves as mothers to the children under their supervision" (Stivers 2002, 60–61). In another case, Sophonia Breckenridge, a resident of Hull House in Chicago, wrote that "economy and efficiency mean something different in their application to public welfare than they do in industry and business" (61).

108   JENNIFER K. ALEXANDER

Much like the settlement house workers of the Progressive era, CBO executive directors and staff brought these early elements of public administration to the partnership. The CBOs were repeatedly referred to as homes for neighborhood residents, conveying the idea of safety and care. They were places where citizens could go for recreation or bring problems and seek resolution. The CBOs had an established history of advocating for neighborhood citizens with public officials that dated as far back as their founding as settlement houses. They were a source of community identity.

F2F revealed the conflict movement, manifest between traditional public administration and the settlement house in the professional orientation of the CWA and CBO social workers. Public agency social work was grounded in procedure, objectivity, expertise, and hierarchy. CBO social workers were embedded in the community, provided services that were based on responsiveness and empathy, and openly advocated for their neighborhoods with the intention of creating better policy. CWA social workers were trained in the medical model of social work, which defines problems at the level of the individual and holds the intent of resolving them through professional assessment, diagnosis, identification of deficiencies, and treatment. The medical model placed CWA social workers in a hierarchical position of experts who make decisions based on what they construe as the relevant facts in a situation and their interpretation of the rules at hand. Combined with the coercive power of the state, this model cast social workers as professional adversaries; those who have the power to coerce or deny agency to others in pursuit of larger social values (Applbaum 1999). Applbaum describes professional adversaries as those who "*act for by acting against*" (1999, 4); in the case of child welfare, *for* children and the public interest *in opposition to* parents who may be negligent or abusive for a variety of reasons.

In contrast, CBO social workers practiced the community-based model of social work, which defines the roots of family challenges in both the individual and the community. Similar to early settlement house reforms, the intention of this perspective is to empower people to solve their own problems through the identification of strengths and skills. Social work practiced as community building requires that CBO social workers understand and relate to the social reality of life in this context and learn to see life as insiders. For this reason, when seeking new employees, CBO executive directors gave preference to qualified applicants who were neighborhood residents.

CBO staff culture minimized hierarchy and the differences between staff and residents. One executive director talked of "leading from behind" as the model for her leadership (Participant interview, 2006). In another instance, we discovered that the CBO staff did not list credentials on their name badges because it created distance in their interactions with community residents.

CBO staff echoed the settlement workers' model of public administration by mediating for citizens in their interactions with the CWA. The F2F partnerships reinforced their capacity to fulfill this role by educating CBO site coordinators and social workers about CWA regulations and procedures. CBO staff members functioned at the intersection of public agency rules and regulations and the reality of children and families in their neighborhoods; they brought their insider perspective to the decision-making process. CBO social workers attended hearings held by CWA social workers with citizens of their neighborhoods, coached families as to their options, and acted as informed witnesses to CWA interactions with families.

Both CBO and CWA social workers recognized that the advocacy and mediation by CBO staff members had altered the interactions between families and the public agency. CWA social workers were accustomed to citizens who had no foundation from which to argue or assert claims on their own behalf because they were unaware of agency rules and how to effectively respond. CBO site coordinators indicated that they were able to help families understand their options and that through coaching, the exchanges between families and CWA social workers became more productive.

Community-based nonprofits understood the importance of their role as a safe haven for the community, and they were careful to guard this identity throughout the partnerships. The objective of community building required that CBOs remain rooted in the neighborhood and not function or appear to function as a proxy for the county. CBO directors maintained their autonomy from the county and alliance with the community by delimiting the extent to which the coercive power of the state could be exercised within the neighborhood centers. Specifically, CBO directors changed the original terms of the partnerships and prohibited "planned visitations" in the neighborhood centers, which are meetings scheduled for children in custody to see their biological parents. CBO directors refused to allow CWA to take custody of any child on their premises. In one case, an executive director refused to allow a social worker to conduct a routine check on a child in day care "because every child in that room knows who the social worker is and it stigmatizes that child." Similarly, an executive director explained that social workers in her CBO support families by *not* participating in meetings with the public agency if the family is not able to attend.

> Sometimes these social workers will try to hold [meetings] during the day and they don't recognize that some of these people can't get off work and come to these meetings without some risk to their employment. Under these circumstances we support holding the meetings at a time when the family can attend. If the family is not at the table, we're not at the table, either.

110   JENNIFER K. ALEXANDER

The final example of how CBOs maintained their alliance with communities was through the establishment of a CBO executive council, a formalized structure that included the executive directors of all CBOs who partnered with CWA in the F2F program. The executive council was created by CBO executive directors when the original F2F liaison, Theresa, left CWA after five years and the CBO executive directors were concerned about how they would make their concerns known to CWA leadership. The executive council represented the interests of all CBOs to the executive director of the CWA, and invited CWA senior staff and the executive director to their meetings.

The Generation and Use of Democratic Knowledge

Settlement house workers were committed to generating scientific knowledge, but they regarded it differently than their bureau men counterparts. They believed that "only what is lived can be understood and translated to others" (Stivers 2002, 97). Early reformers believed that the data they carefully recorded, documenting the experiences of people in urban poverty, would serve as a catalyst for generating responsive policy and, ultimately, social progress. The interpretation of these facts and even the discernment of relevant facts to document was the foundation of democratic knowledge. Similarly, John Dewey (1927) argued that democratic knowledge is generated from an inclusive dialogue intended to discern what the facts in a situation mean. "Trustworthy, accurate knowledge comes from tangible familiarity and developing the capacity to see things from the inside" (Stivers 2002, 96).

The F2F partnerships fostered democratic knowledge by assigning CWA social workers to the CBOs where agency tasks were integrated with the work of CBO social workers. CWA social workers were oriented to the neighborhoods by CBO staff. They learned the social reality of the citizens they served, the businesses and services that existed in the neighborhood, the foster parents, and of various people who lived there. One CWA social worker remarked that she was stunned to learn of the paucity of services available to residents; there was no bank or ATM located within a few miles of her assigned neighborhood center.

A shared understanding of the problem of child welfare emerged as CWA and CBO social workers were required to integrate tasks. In the early years of the partnerships, they did not have the same definition of the problem. But in the course of sharing information and solving problems together, both sides shifted their perspective and came to define the situation of children in their neighborhoods in a new light. CBO staff members were surprised to learn the actual number of children that had been removed from their communities and the reasons why. As the caseloads of CWA social workers were confined to a particular neighborhood, public agency staff developed "tangible familiarity" with the experiences of the people they served through ongoing information exchange and stronger working relationships.

County social workers indicated that initially the work in partnership was exceedingly difficult. CWA social workers were reticent about sharing information with the CBO staff and families. After functioning as "experts in charge," they felt a loss of control over their work. "We were shoe horned in [to working with the neighborhood centers] but over time we came to realize how much the partnerships helped with our work" (participant interview, 2008). Another social worker noted,

> At the start we saw a lot of risk because we were revealing what CWA had not been particularly adept at and we were afraid we would lose control over the cases. We later realized that it was largely a perceived risk because most of what we were sharing [with CBO social workers] was already known. (Participant interview, 2008)

Democratic knowledge generated in the CBOs informed decisions regarding high-risk families and their children. Previous to F2F, a decision as to whether to take custody of a child or how to best respond to a case of neglect or abuse was made by an individual social worker. As with most frontline public administration, the framework for decisions is highly rule infused but social workers remain in the position to make policy through their decisions, "governing through their values, interpretations of rule and procedure" with considerable discretion and little immediate oversight (Smith and Lipsky 1993, 116). With the advent of F2F, most family-related decisions and those that pertained to custody were shifted to team decision meetings (TDMs) held at the CBO. These open meetings included the county social worker, the CBO social worker, and any individuals the family members might ask to speak on their behalf. The F2F model required that decisions regarding the welfare of a child be made in an open discussion intended to review the relevant facts, interpret their meaning, and identify what practical solutions would best support the safety of the child and the health of the family. While the authority for final decisions remained with the county social workers, the discussion and interpretation of the relevant facts was inclusive and open.

TDMs resulted in a more open and forthright dialogue because they empowered citizens in several respects. The meetings provided a foundation for citizens to present their experiences to people who knew them and could knowledgeably advocate on their behalf. Judgments that emerged from TDMs were informed by the intimate knowledge of several people engaged in identifying practical solutions to a problem, rather than a lone public servant saddled with a heavy caseload and limited information. The result was that TDMs were a vehicle for agency accountability with their service population that was in stark contrast to past practice. Prior to F2F, the CWA was not accountable to parents or family members in the clearest sense of accounting, the giving of reasons for decisions based in a shared value system (Friedrich 1958). CWA authority rested in their expertise, a professional interpretation of the facts in a situation, and the coercive power of the state. A CWA social worker had the authority to take a child into custody for reasons that resonated with the agency alone, the agency was under no obligation to tell the biological parent where the child was going or when the child would be back. F2F created a public agency decision process grounded in democratic knowledge, where social workers provided reasons for their decisions that reflected not only agency rules but a shared interpretation of facts resulting from the dialogue.

The Responsibilities of Administrators

If public administration is a practical endeavor of problem solving that occurs among public servants and citizens, if it requires public space, a community home where people join together to speak about community concerns and hear what each believes to be the truth (Stivers 2008), then what are the responsibilities of public administrators? Scholars who support democratic governance have argued that administrators no longer act as experts who inform and decide, but as public servants who act in horizontal relationships with citizens to develop practical knowledge of their experience and approach solutions pragmatically (Cooper 1998; Denhardt and Denhardt 2000; Alexander and Nank 2009). This requires a shift in focus from procedural concerns to a mindfulness about the purpose of action. Administrators need to be equipped with facilitative skills, the ability to actively listen, manage conflict, foster dialogue, and construct solutions that align with citizen perspectives and needs.

In the practical application, CWA social workers repeatedly indicated that making the transition from expert to an engaged public servant was arduous. At the inception of the study, mid-level leadership and frontline social workers were resistant to sharing responsibility for child welfare with a community represented by CBOs. They questioned whether the agency leadership was committed to F2F. They expressed a loss of power that resulted from the sharing of information with citizens and CBO social workers. CWA social workers struggled with the difficulty of reasoning with others and providing reasons that made sense to the people involved rather than falling back on the rules. They recognized the shift of power that had occurred as licensed CBO social workers acted as family advocates. Decision making in open meetings created a new form of agency accountability.

The continued support of F2F through four changes in agency director-ships between 1998 and 2002 and an agency turnover rate that exceeded 25 percent left remaining social workers with little recourse but to disperse to their geographically assigned CBO and find a way to make it work. As the partnerships with the CBOs took on momentum and normalized, CWA staff realized they were making more sound decisions. When we returned to the study in 2007, county social workers told us that the ongoing practice of team decision meetings had changed the nature of their work. They were experiencing the tangible gains of partnering; social workers had more information on which to base decisions, and the final judgments reflected a number of perspectives rather than a single one. CWA social workers felt less risk for the decisions they made because responsibility for discerning right action was shared and they had come to trust the judgment of their CBO partners. One CWA social worker noted,

> When I was 23 years old with a graduate degree and not much life experience beyond my Catholic suburban upbringing, I could stand in a family's door and tell them I was taking their kids and that was that. By the same token, if I decided the situation was not that dire and a child died, I lived with that decision alone. Today it's a whole lot different.

CWA social workers had to learn new skills to support their new way of functioning in partnership—how to facilitate meetings by listening, managing conflict, and fostering an inclusive dialogue. When the policy of holding open hearings was instituted, social workers felt exposed and under pressure to explain the basis of their decisions while they were in the process of forming them. At first, they would leave the room and formulate an agency position while the family and CBO social workers awaited their return. CBO executive directors objected and pointed out that although the final decision remained with the county social worker, the original terms of the partnership were that discussions and interpretations of facts would occur as an open dialogue. With this objection noted, the CWA executive director supported the CBO's and informed social workers that they would "have to find a way to stay in their chairs" and come to a decision they could support (Participant interview 2008). The rules of TDMs continue to evolve in response to new situations with families, and the agency remains committed to working out decisions that serve families, through open dialogue.

Conclusion

This unusual case of a public-nonprofit partnership demonstrates how a public human services agency that was caught in a mission crisis and confined

114   JENNIFER K. ALEXANDER

by bureaucratic proceduralism and plummeting morale found its way to solid ground by embracing an interactive practice of democratic governance through partnerships with community-based organizations. The national effort to systematically change child welfare to a preventive, community-based approach has been evaluated countless times, most often by schools of social work and the participating counties themselves. F2F is a success story that has yet to make its way into the public administration literature. But it is a hopeful story and tangible evidence that democratic governance is a viable method of healing the problem of governance failure and creating a sense on the part of citizens that responsible and capable behavior is forthcoming, that government is, indeed, accountable to the citizens it serves.

The structure of the F2F partnerships and their outcomes were not intentionally related to the ongoing dialogue in public administration on how we should proceed in practice: efficient public management devoted to technique and procedure or caring and responsive governance in pursuit of mutually defined ends. It was intended to improve the capacity of communities to respond to their own high-risk families and children at risk for abuse, and to ensure the safety and healthy development of children who were removed from their homes by the administrative state. By most measures, this was achieved. Data revealed that between 2000 and 2010, the number of children taken into custody dropped from 6,000 to 1,600. The number of children who are able to stay at home or with a family member through supportive services increased, the number placed in institutional or group facilities decreased, and the resolution of cases progresses more quickly. Unfortunately, the number of placements with resource families in the neighborhoods has not been as successful as hoped, as only a fifth of the children taken into custody are placed with foster families in their neighborhoods. Children of color continue to be disproportionately represented in caseloads (65 percent). But no longer are there reports of children languishing in the CWA lobby for days, left there by foster parents, social service agencies, or biological parents. No longer is the agency pelted by the local press with accusations of incompetence or calls for a state takeover by county commissioners.

The untold story of F2F is how partnerships with mediating institutions can link the public sector with citizens, provide a safe forum and foundation for dialogue, foster the generation of democratic knowledge that informs administrative decision making, and deliver responsive and caring services to citizens. There is much to gain from a collaborative and caring approach to human problems. Indeed, partnerships that foster democratic governance have expanded our definition of "what government can properly and successfully do" (Wilson [1887] 1987) and how we might do those proper things in a new and better way.

References

Alexander, Jennifer. 1997. "Avoiding the Issue: Racism and Administrative Responsibility in Public Administration." *American Review of Public Administration* 27 (4): 343–61.

Alexander, Jennifer, and Renee Nank. 2009. "Public-Nonprofit Partnerships: Realizing the New Public Service." *Administration & Society* 41 (3): 364–86.

American Humane Association. 1998. *A Comprehensive Review of the XXXX County Department of Children and Family Services.* Englewood, CO: Author.

Annie E. Casey Foundation. 1997. *City Kids Count: Data on the Well-Being of Children in Large Cities.* Baltimore, MD: Author.

Applbaum, Arthur. 1999. *Ethics for Adversaries: The Morality of Roles in Public and Professional Life.* Princeton, NJ: Princeton University Press.

Box, Richard C. 1998. *Citizen Governance.* Thousand Oaks, CA: Sage.

Cooper, Terry. 1991. *An Ethic of Citizenship for Public Administration.* Englewood Cliffs, NJ: Prentice-Hall.

———. 1998. *The Responsible Administrator.* San Francisco: Jossey-Bass.

DeMuro, Paul. 1995. "Family to Family Tools for Rebuilding Foster Care: Building Partnerships with Neighborhoods and Local Communities." Baltimore, MD: Annie E. Casey Foundation.

Denhardt, Janet V., and Robert B. Denhardt. 2007. *The New Public Service: Serving, not Steering.* Exp. ed. Armonk: M.E. Sharpe.

Denhardt, Robert B., and Janet V. Denhardt. 2000. "The New Public Service: Serving Rather Than Steering." *Public Administration Review* 60 (6): 449–59.

Dewey, John. 1927. *The Public and Its Problems.* New York: Holt.

Flyvbjerg, Bent. 2004. "Five Misunderstandings about Case Study Research." *Qualitative Inquiry* 12 (2): 219–45.

Frederickson, H. George. 1997. *The Spirit of Public Administration.* San Francisco: Jossey-Bass.

Frederickson, H. George, and R. Chandler. 1984. "A Symposium on Citizenship and Public Administration." *Public Administration Review* 44: 99–206.

Friedrich, Carl J. (ed.) 1958. *Authority* (Nomos 1). Cambridge, MA: Harvard University Press.

Kantor, Rosabeth Moss. 1972. *Commitment and Community.* Cambridge, MA: Harvard University Press.

King, Cheryl S., Camilla Stivers, and Collaborators (1998). *Government Is Us: Strategies for an Anti-government Era.* Thousand Oaks, CA: Sage.

Sandel, M., 1981. *Liberalism and the Limits of Justice.* Cambridge, MA: Cambridge University Press.

Smith, Steven, and Michael Lipsky. 1993. *Nonprofits for Hire.* Cambridge. MA: Harvard University Press.

Stivers, Camilla. 2000. "Citizenship Ethics in Public Administration" In *Handbook of Administrative Ethics,* ed. Terry Cooper, 583–602. New York: Marcel Dekker.

———. 2002. *Bureau Men, Settlement Women: Constructing Public Administration in the Progressive Era.* Lawrence: University Press of Kansas.

———. 2008. *Governance in Dark Times.* Washington, DC: Georgetown University Press.

Wilson, Woodrow. (1887) 1987. "The Study of Administration." In *Classics of Public Administration,* 2d ed., ed. Jay Shafritz and Albert Hyde. Chicago: Dorsey Press.

Wolin, Sheldon. 1994. "Contract and Birthright." In *Communitarianism: A New Public Ethics,* ed. Markate Daly. Belmont, CA: ITP Wadsworth.

Part III

Stories of Practice

The chapters in Part III provide rich stories of engagement in practice. What these stories reveal is that working to bring more citizens into administrative processes is much more than simply (not that this is simple) setting up and facilitating participatory processes. We also have to completely rethink institutional practices, how agencies are organized, and how we interact with each other, let alone our interactions with citizens. The path to deeper engagement has many routes, as these chapters show. We cannot have an ideal of deeper engagement as long as our institutions practice institutional racism—addressing institutional racism is a path or a portal to deeper engagement. We cannot have an ideal of deeper engagement if we are not practicing more social and environmental justice. Sustainability efforts, while apparently about being "green," are also portals to deeper engagement because they require that we rethink our relationships among ourselves and our environments and that we practice environmental, social, and economic justice. Finally, we cannot be politically naïve when we seek to change our organizations and practices—we have to expect that the road to elsewhere will be pretty bumpy.

Walt Kovalick, Alan Walts, and Suzanne Wells revive and revise Kovalick and Kelly's chapter in the first edition. Kovalick, Walts, and Wells tell of the bumpy road the U.S. Environmental Protection Agency (EPA) has been on and the ways in which programs, approaches, and models of participation and engagement have evolved over time, leading to the more activist and collaborative model the EPA is currently developing. All of this is in the face of increasingly complicated, large-scale environmental problems (e.g., climate change); a huge organization with regulatory, as well as facilitative, responsibilities; a more robust and active environmental justice movement; and the "game-changing" (page 120) impact of new information technology. All of these increasingly level the playing field for opening dialogue and what the authors call "authentic engagement," which involves "'curiosity' regarding the information and experiences of others" (Ibid.).

Claire Mostel tells the touching tale of the death of a much-loved and valued citizen-centered organization of Miami-Dade county. With dark humor she describes the passing:

> Residents of unincorporated Miami-Dade county are mourning the death of Team Metro. The county department that put a face on local government

passed away on September 30, 2008. It is survived by loyal staff members and county residents who appreciated having a government office in their neighborhood (page 147).

Her story is a cautionary tale about an organization that had a "glorious fourteen-year run of providing excellent customer service" (page 147). The cause of death was "rumored to be politics and budget cuts" (Ibid.). Her story encompasses an "autopsy" in which she reflects on the causes of the passing of the organization and posits lessons learned that may apply in other situations.

Elliott Bronstein, Glenn Harris, Ron Harris-White, and Julie Nelson tell the story of the Race and Social Justice Initiative (RSJI) of the City of Seattle. This initiative, a mandate of former mayor Greg Nichols, seeks to address racism within city organizations and also within the community. A case study of Seattle Public Utilities' (SPU) implementation of RSJI is presented, with evidence of how SPU successfully achieved the intended ends of workforce and economic equity, improving services for immigrant and refugee communities, public engagement, capacity building, and changes in business practices. The city is now working to implement RSJI in the larger community. Their story shows how an initiative geared toward addressing social and economic justice issues is a portal to deeper engagement with citizens and to better possibilities for the future. The story also shows how such an initiative can be politically successful (it helps that it was the mayor's mandate), in contrast to the Miami-Dade story.

Michael Mucha describes a case of transformational change: the implementation of sustainability practices in the City of Olympia. He tells the story of organizational change in the Department of Public Works and shows how sustainability efforts, coupled with the design and implementation of an organizational, cultural, and management strategy with sustainability as a central organizational and managerial principle, can go beyond simply being "green." He presents the Sustainable Action Map (SAM), a decision-making tool being used citywide (and adopted by many cities and other organizations around the world). Sustainability efforts, if they are practiced as a system-wide movement to change organizations and behaviors, have the potential to, as he says, "restore and renew relationships among and between citizens and their governments—we might even begin trusting each other again" (page 175).

And last (but not least), Larry Luton weaves a tangled web in his fictional account of a sustainability task force and the city's sustainability coordinator, Jason Allen. All of the political, social, and organizational machinations nodded to in previous stories are detailed here in Jason's journey from eager facilitator of a change process to brow-beaten administrator hoping to eke out something positive for his efforts. Luton's tale is cautionary and educational, not to mention a breath of fresh, fictional air.

8

The EPA Seeks Its Role in Communities

Evolutionary Engagement

Walter W. Kovalick Jr., Alan Walts, and Suzanne Wells

Almost fifteen years have passed since the original authors wrote this chapter describing the organizational and policy evolution of the U.S. Environmental Protection Agency's (EPA's) work engaging members of the public. The new team of authors notes with sadness the passing of Margaret Kelly, who shaped the first edition. She would agree, however, that even then the story was only partially complete. The EPA continues to benefit from and respond to both internal and external factors in designing and carrying out its public participation, community involvement, and collaborative problem-solving work. These range from new pressures from communities and members of the public; to developments in the profession of public participation; to the evolution of the EPA's own programs, the approaches they use, and their models for community involvement.

This revised chapter presents some of the most influential changes and discusses the increasingly activist and collaborative model for the EPA's community involvement activities.

First, the chapter identifies several additional early policy anchors and seminal publications that altered the landscape of the EPA's community involvement work. Also, we have made a more complete accounting of the statutes and regulations that drive the EPA's work—then and now.

Second, moving beyond traditional pollution problems, NIMBY issues, and questions about new chemicals from the 1990s, the context for community involvement at the local level has expanded to the national level. Large-scale, increasingly complicated issues with broad environmental, economic, and social implications have come to the fore in the last decade, leading to elevated public awareness, concern, and sophistication about environmental issues.

120   WALTER W. KOVALICK JR., ALAN WALTS, AND SUZANNE WELLS

These include climate change, water quality and quantity, new materials (e.g., nanotechnologies) with often-uncertain environmental and health impacts, and increasing attention on how environmental protection relates to community development. Our new approaches are evolving with this new context in mind.

Third, and of particular note in this edition, is a more robust treatment of the advent and ongoing maturation of the environmental justice movement. Attention to how effectively the EPA's regulations and activities protect vulnerable and disadvantaged communities, together with developments in our scientific capacity to evaluate stressors across ecosystems and communities, are leading the EPA to recalibrate its approach toward protecting human health and the environment.

Fourth, this edition offers a more informed and sophisticated model for the EPA's approach to community involvement. The EPA seeks to involve communities in both regulatory activities and joint stewardship efforts. This evolved model moves beyond the more clinical and neutral convener suggested in the first edition, toward one that recognizes new approaches to bringing stakeholders' valuable insights and information into the decision-making process. We suggest that a richer view of collaboration better describes these evolving approaches—one that involves authentic engagement and "curiosity" regarding the information and experiences of others.

Finally, embedded in this chapter (and obvious to all) is the game-changing impact of new information technology. The arrival of the Internet, search engines, and social media (blogs, wikis, Facebook, Twitter, and so on) has dramatically increased public access to detailed information at desks and kitchen tables across America. These technological changes have enhanced and accelerated the availability of information about the nation's environmental health—much of it (but by no means all) collected and made available by the EPA. The Internet is a significant source of empowerment and an organizing tool for communities, although socioeconomic factors still influence access to and use of information.[1] While information itself does not solve the puzzle of effective community involvement, we believe it will increasingly level the playing field for opening dialogues and authentic engagement.

This edition adds two new authors with national and regional experience in working with communities. We trust that it more faithfully recounts the legacy of past community involvement approaches at the EPA and captures the current and future directions as we try to continuously improve our engagement with the EPA's many publics and stakeholders.

The EPA and the Public

Few federal agencies have as much direct impact on the public as the EPA. The air we breathe and water we drink, the insecticides and chemicals we use and are exposed to, the automobiles we drive, the fruits and vegetables we eat, and the gas stations and waste sites that need cleaning up are all affected by decisions made by the agency. Reflecting on our experiences as practitioners in a federal regulatory agency, we see several important influences and forces that shape the nature of this agency's interaction with the public.

We believe a complex set of factors influence how the agency has structured and developed its interactions with communities. While some of these factors may be common to all public institutions, some strike us as unique to the kind of public administration carried out at the EPA. We explore three themes in this chapter as a basis for our characterization of how the EPA engages the public at the most local level. First, the nature of public health and environmental protection has become more complex, less obvious in its impact, and more controversial over the last forty years. Second, the EPA's organizational arrangements and policy commitments to engage the public have changed and adapted over the same period in order to adjust to the increasing needs for relationships with many different sectors of society. Third, the mandates presented to the EPA—largely through legislation, but also from other authoritative sources—have caused it to adapt its program implementation strategies and, more specifically, its efforts to engage with public groups and individuals. Using a variety of organizational arrangements and program mechanisms, EPA practitioners have sought approaches to improve the level of engagement with the individuals and communities that EPA programs affect. In the first edition of this book, this chapter described the EPA's newly evolved role as that of a "task-oriented, but inclusive and balanced convener." This evolution has continued, fueled by the dynamic tension between centralized expertise and shared responsibility that was present at the inception of the EPA. That emerging role is inextricably bound up with the concept of governance based on "environmental stewardship" as well as regulatory authority. The EPA defines *environmental stewardship* as the responsibility for environmental quality shared by all those whose actions affect the environment. The dimensions of meaning of this concept have been articulated and are now being explored by the National Advisory Council for Environmental Policy and Technology (NACEPT).[2] Its implications for approaches to community involvement are discussed next.

Environmental Protection—Then and Now

Twenty million people celebrated the first Earth Day in 1970. In the same year, President Nixon created the EPA to bring scattered "research, monitoring, standard-setting and enforcement activities" within a single agency, recognizing that "for pollution control purposes the environment must be perceived as a single, interrelated system" (U.S. EPA 1970). Despite this purpose of centralizing expertise and authority, from the start one of the agency's principal roles was "[a]ssisting others, through grants, technical assistance and other means in arresting pollution of the environment" (Ibid.). The EPA declared that it must be an advocate, not simply a regulator and researcher: "As we work toward pollution abatement, we shall also strive to provide information and leadership; to enhance the environmental awareness of all the people and all of the institutions of this society."[3]

This role was widely accepted at the time, as the first administrator, William Ruckelshaus, and his immediate successor, Russell Train, were faced with gross examples of environmental pollution. The Clean Air Act and Clean Water Act were directed at air and surface water pollution problems that were visible and understood by the public. Further, the EPA had been given the tools to address these problems and was prepared to use them. Administrator Ruckelshaus believed it was important to establish the serious intent of the EPA's enforcement arm and undertook a series of important, public enforcement actions against corporate and municipal entities (U.S. EPA 1993).

But, despite the EPA's ongoing commitment to regulation and enforcement, public attitudes soon shifted to a mixture of cautious trust, dissatisfaction, and, at times, suspicion. These shifts mainly reflect an ongoing tension between two of the EPA's roles since its genesis: that of acting as the center of expertise and authority, and that of assisting others in achieving shared environmental protection goals. Factors shaping changes in public attitudes and exacerbating the tension between these roles include increasing attention to environmental and economic tradeoffs (and less accessible, more technical analysis of these tradeoffs in rule making); increasingly specialized and opaque approaches to identifying and managing environmental risk; an enforcement approach that is often based on compliance with prescribed technological standards at particular facilities rather than directly with area-wide standards of environmental quality or health; and a perception by affected communities that the EPA is unresponsive to, or does not have the regulatory authority to address their most salient environmental and health concerns.

Environmental Protection and Economics

The 1970s and 1980s were times of significant societal change in the legal and policy environment surrounding the EPA. Along with new worker and consumer protection statutes, several new environmental protection statutes were enacted, including the Clean Air Act, the Clean Water Act, the Toxic

Substances Control Act, the Resource Conservation and Recovery Act, and the Comprehensive Environmental Response, Compensation, and Liability Act (CERCLA, or Superfund). Capital investments and operating expenditures necessary to comply with many new environmental regulations, including pollution control or treatment technology, had to compete with other investments that corporations wanted to make. Concern was raised about stringent regulations and their resulting costs. In its role as a regulatory agency, the EPA had incorporated cost-benefit considerations in developing many of its rules (although consideration of costs was less explicit in certain environmental statutes). However, during this period several succeeding administrations emphasized cost considerations and economic impact analysis. Since that time, such analysis has become increasingly important (U.S. Office of Management and Budget 1996). The EPA's role in striking the right balance between costs and benefits remains contentious (U.S. Supreme Court 2009) and may have contributed to its diminished image as an "advocate" for the environment.

More Complicated Challenges and Approaches to Determining Harm

Successful implementation of regulatory programs under these new statutes brought gross pollution problems under control, or at least mitigated the most visible and significant impacts (such as emissions from large industrial sources and automobiles, poor visibility in national parks, and toxic and flammable chemical releases to rivers). Technology rose to meet the challenge of environmental regulations as attention shifted to less evident impacts. New and improved detection devices enabled regulatory agencies and industry to detect minute amounts of toxic pollutants in air, water, soil, and food. This capacity led some citizens to believe that any detectable amount was a hazard to public health.

Together with its increased detection capacity, the EPA also began to use more complex analytical tools, such as computer models, to evaluate health and ecological impacts. The concept of risk assessment was introduced as a scientifically credible expression of potential harm, along with explicit recognition of the uncertainties in such assessments due to a variety of reasons (e.g., the quality of the data itself, the effects of chemicals on animals as differentiated from humans, and the nature of exposure; National Research Council 1983; U.S. EPA 1990). Scientists used risk assessment tools and models to identify prospective risks associated with diverse industry practices. Characterization of these risks then supported development of new (and increasingly complex) rules. The sheer number of industrial and municipal facilities also made modeling necessary because it was often impossible for the EPA or state regulatory agencies to isolate and assess risk on a source-specific basis.

The change in the environmental protection mission from removing visible assaults on the air and water to risk management using risk assessments that may include consideration of costs and benefits is not widely understood by the general public (National Research Council 1994). The EPA was not always able to explain in an understandable way to the general public the relative significance of exposure to small amounts of chemicals and pollutants, adding to the public feeling that the agency was not protecting their health. Further, experts disagree as to the appropriate characterization of health and ecological benefits and costs. These complexities have caused some constituencies to view EPA decisions more skeptically, and some have questioned risk assessment itself on environmental justice grounds (Kuehn 1996).

Others, including the EPA's National Environmental Justice Advisory Council (NEJAC) (NEJAC 2004), have argued that the EPA must conduct even more complex analyses that consider the cumulative impacts of multiple stressors on a given population or community. Public interest in and awareness of the health impacts of environmental chemical exposures and their interactions with other stressors continue to grow as more information is assembled about exposure to multiple chemicals in air, water, and soil from different sources. The EPA has responded to these increasing requests for ways to understand and evaluate combined impacts. The agency's Framework for Cumulative Risk Assessment defines the general concepts and considerations for these assessments (U.S. EPA 2003a), building on earlier work on planning and scoping of cumulative risk assessments (U.S. EPA 1997b). The agency has gained significant experience and continues to improve its understanding of how to plan for and conduct such assessments (U.S. EPA 2007). However, the technical and resource challenges remain significant, and cumulative risk assessment is a far less settled area of scientific work than the quantitative risk assessments previously discussed.

In addition to the technical challenges, there are challenges related to the scope of the EPA's regulatory authority. Existing regulatory regimes do not consider cumulative impacts across media (i.e., air, water, soil) or even within media in a defined geographical area. This means that there is little routine collection and evaluation of evidence to know whether or not the population is protected from real-world effects of cumulative environmental stressors. For example, the Resource Conservation and Recovery Act required permits for treatment, storage, and disposal methods for hazardous waste. These permits apply to individual facilities, and cumulative effects from other facilities are not generally considered. Thus, if a second facility in a community applies for a permit, the application will not be considered in the context of other facilities and the pollution allowed by their respective permits. Permits do not, therefore, consider cumulative risk in a community. Indeed, if an industrial facility manages to reduce emissions of air pollutants through process or other operational changes, it may then increase production volume until subsequent emissions increase again to the levels allowed in their permit.

In fact, monitoring programs established through regulations are generally targeted at measuring whether the industrial process is in compliance with applicable regulations and permits, not health impacts resulting from industrial operations. An exception to this is the notice given to localities of high ozone levels and subsequent directives to sensitive individuals. Although the agency has made some progress over the years in measuring "indicators" of environmental improvement, it still largely enforces compliance with regulations based on a technology standard, process measure, or risk assessment. These approaches cannot effectively consider and address the health effects in an affected community resulting from cumulative and aggregate sources of exposure to pollution, due to both scientific and regulatory challenges. For example, because permitting reviews independently evaluate each permitted facility and its emissions—irrespective of its location adjacent to other industrial or pollution control facilities—this gave rise to concerns about the undue impact of multiple permitted facilities on communities of lower socioeconomic status. Advances in developing index-based approaches to community-based risk assessment, as part of collaborative problem-solving efforts with meaningful community involvement, provide one way to meet these concerns despite limits to technical capacity and regulatory authority (Zartarian and Schultz 2009; Medina-Vera et al. 2010).

More Citizen Engagement in Environmental Decision Making

An engaged citizenry is essential to environmental protection and to pushing the government to go further than it might go on its own. There has been a continued, and increasingly sophisticated, presence of community-based organizations working to engage and support involvement of community members in environmental issues. For example, Lois Gibbs, who had lived at Love Canal, the site near Niagara Falls, New York, that spurred the passage of CERCLA, founded the Citizens Clearinghouse for Hazardous Waste in 1981, which is now called the Center for Health, Environment & Justice (CHEJ). The mission of CHEJ is to provide technical and organizational assistance to individuals and communities facing toxic hazards. Another example is the Center for Public Environmental Oversight (CPEO), an organization formed in 1992 that promotes and facilitates public participation in the oversight of environmental activities at hazardous waste sites.

The ongoing presence of these nonprofit organizations demonstrates a recognition that individuals in communities are often the eyes and ears of government agencies—bringing issues to the attention of local, state, and federal agencies, working collaboratively with these agencies to solve problems, and, in some cases, pressing government agencies to go further than they might otherwise go. While the EPA can and should respond to information that can be considered under its regulatory authority, these responses may be insufficient to address community concerns. One example of this is permitting the Waste Technologies Industries incinerator in East Liverpool, Ohio, to be located near a public school and a residential neighborhood. This situation, and dissatisfaction with environmental authorities, prompted the emergence of local grassroots activism to oppose the granting of a permit for an incinerator at that site. Further, local activists filed citizen suits to prevent the incinerator from operating (U.S. Government Accountability Office 1994).

In another instance, an industrial release in clear violation of environmental permits caused an outcry among neighboring communities in Contra Costa County, California. Enforcement and response actions by regulatory agencies did not satisfy the citizens. Organized community activism emerged, obtaining a monetary settlement for the citizens and an innovative agreement on the part of the facility to partner with the community to provide access to information, inspections, and independent technical assistance (Hallissy 1997). Affected communities are demanding and obtaining the capacity to appraise on their own the sustainability of industrial facilities, in a manner that goes far beyond what the EPA may (or can) require of a facility under the law.

Another instance of community opposition is the response to federal and state permits allowing Chemical Waste Management, Inc., to store and dispose of polychlorinated biphenyl waste at the Kettleman Hills facility in Kings County, California (Yamashita 2009). The EPA completed an extensive draft of its environmental justice assessment at this site and has taken other steps to consider impacts and community concerns.[4]

In some cases, citizen activism achieves its aims despite limits to the EPA's authority. An example is that of Shintech, a polyvinyl chloride facility proposed for construction in Convent, Louisiana, in 1996. Following two years of opposition, the facility withdrew its permit application in September 1998. This was viewed as a major victory against environmental injustice, driven by citizen opposition to the facility (Environmental Justice Resource Center. (Undated). Before the facility's withdrawal, citizen groups were also successful in their requests for EPA action, including initiating an investigation under Title VI of the Civil Rights Act of 1964. Initial results from this investigation were used by citizen groups to support their opposition (Louisiana Environmental Action Network, April 7, 2004).

Box 8.1
Collaborating to Solve Problems

For decades, the local industries near Torrance, California, released DDT, PCBs, and other chemicals into the sewer system, which emptied into the ocean off the Palos Verdes Peninsula. Studies showed elevated levels of the chemicals DDT and PCB in the ocean sediment and in the fish living there. In 1997, the U.S. EPA proposed the Palos Verdes Shelf site on the Superfund National Priorities List. The remedy chosen for the site involved capping the ocean sediments to minimize exposure. Over time, the capping remedy is expected to reduce harmful exposure to contaminants. However, in the near term, people who regularly eat fish caught near the contaminated area face greater health risks because of prolonged exposure to toxic chemicals. In order to address the risks posed by the site from eating contaminated fish, California placed restrictions near the Palos Verdes Shelf on commercial and recreational fishing. In 2003, U.S. EPA established and funded the Fish Contamination Education Collaborative (FCEC) to educate the public on the health risks posed by eating chemically contaminated fish and to encourage the public to adopt safer fish consumption practices.

The FCEC is comprised of several local nonprofit organizations and key individuals with strong ties to the local community. The area near the Palos Verdes Shelf is an area rich in cultural diversity, and it is comprised of over nine ethnic and national groups. Nonprofit organizations Heal the Bay, Boat People SOS, St. Anselm's, and Cabrillo Marine Aquarium were involved, as well as individuals.

The FCEC worked to effectively communicate with the public about the risk associated with the consumption of contaminated fish. The Family and Community Outreach program interacts with the community by giving presentations at schools, English as a second language classes, and health fairs. St. Anselm's and Boat People SOS, an organization within the Vietnamese community, educate members about the risk of consuming contaminated fish. The FCEC created a Web site (www.pvsfish.org) to help inform the community about where to fish, and proper ways to prepare fish that include removing fatty portions to lower the amount of chemicals consumed. FCEC educates more than 10,000 anglers each year and disseminates information to thirty different bait shops and fishing supply stores near the piers. The outreach activities have been conducted in approximately fourteen languages to better communicate with citizens. This has had positive results.

Often, because of limited staff or cultural misunderstandings, the government's efforts to implement a fish advisory consists of posting fish advisory signs or publishing general fish advisory pamphlets. The effort at the Palos Verdes Shelf is an example of communities taking more ownership of the environmental problems they face and working constructively together with the government to conduct more effective outreach activities than the government could have conducted on its own.

Organizational and Policy Development

While these changes in the nature of the EPA's work were going on, the institution itself was adjusting and adapting its organizational structure to better recognize and collaborate with its numerous and diverse publics—including members of the public as individuals. In reviewing the changes in this structure, together with significant developments in policy, we see some pointers to the EPA's evolving role as the convener of interested parties. Several significant aspects of these organizational changes are the continuous change and adaptation during several administrations, the maturing of the organizational role from public "affairs" to "involvement" or "engagement" with an added educational component, the growing number of named constituencies with an organizational focus, and the creation of organizational entities tied to underrepresented stakeholder groups. What we will see during this review is that despite numerous adaptations and positive efforts to touch members of the public as individuals, a federal agency must primarily use recognized groups or communities to interact on national issues. Recent efforts to define underrepresented populations and then seek to define and respond to their interests are works in progress.

Formed in 1970 through an amalgamation of a number of programs across the federal departments, the EPA's suborganization to engage the public began as a traditional Office of Public Affairs nestled comfortably with numerous other functional offices reporting to the administrator. A citizen information division came (and went) as part of this office between 1972 and 1977, along with the advent of a visitor center and an information center. In these early years, one sees in the organizational structure the "standard" approach used by many federal agencies. The use of the term "public affairs" implies the simple transactions between the agency and members of the public. Information is disseminated as necessary, and requests are fulfilled when made. Of course, an early, important function included interaction with the press on the EPA's business. In 1978, during the Carter administration, the Office of Public Awareness became the new moniker, with a specific media services organization cited on the organization charts. Again, the choice of the word *awareness* began to imply a different kind of responsibility and relationship than transaction management and information dissemination. Further, in 1980, a separate and equal Office of Press Services was created. Presumably, this was a signal of equivalent attention devoted to raising the sensitivities of the public and to keeping the press up to date.

On January 19, 1981, the last day of the Carter administration, the EPA issued its first policy on public participation, which remained in place for almost two decades. The purpose of the policy was "to strengthen EPA's commitment to public participation and establish uniform procedures for participation by the public in EPA's decision-making process" (U.S. Government 1981). The policy identified five functions that must be carried out to ensure effective public participation:

1. *Identification:* The need to identify groups or members of the public who may be interested in or affected by a forthcoming action.
2. *Outreach:* The need for the agency to make sure the public receives adequate, timely information concerning a forthcoming action or decision.
3. *Dialogue:* There must be dialogue between officials responsible for a forthcoming action or decision and the interested and affected members of the public.
4. *Assimilation:* The agency must demonstrate in its decisions and actions that it has understood and fully considered public comments.
5. *Feedback:* The agency must provide feedback to participants and interested parties concerning the outcome of the public's involvement.

Beginning in 1981, during the Reagan administration, the public's "office" went back to being the Office of Public Affairs, again subsuming the press functions within it. William Ruckelshaus, returning to lead the EPA for a second time starting in 1983, established a so-called government-in-a-fishbowl policy. This was a reaction to the brief tenure of the previous administrative team, which had been accused of holding meetings with corporate representatives behind closed doors. The net result was a more determined effort to make the "public's business" more open through such mechanisms as making the calendars of senior officials available, better documentation of interactions with advocates on any side of rule making, and a more open approach to supplying nonconfidential information requested by the public.

In 1984 came the first elevation of external affairs for the agency, creating an assistant administrator for external affairs, a presidential appointment confirmed by the U.S. Senate. Grouped under this presidentially appointed political official were offices of congressional relations, federal activities, intergovernmental relations, legislation, and public affairs. At this juncture, the agency was grouping all of its relations management under a senior political official. In one sense, it meant that relating to these publics—Congress, federal agencies, states, tribes, and cities, and the press and the general public—was important enough business to garner the use of a scarce presidential appointment. From another perspective, the EPA had begun to parse up the general public into subgroups for more focused attention, with community members being one group among many. In 1985 some additional changes were made with an Office of Public and Private Liaison substituted for the previous Office of Intergovernmental Relations and a new community relations division formed. Here we see the first organizational manifestation of a need to relate to the public as individuals within communities—not via the press or their other surrogates.

In 1986 some further shifts were made to create an Office of Community and Intergovernmental Liaison in parallel with the Office of Public Affairs. Here we see "communities" being linked with cities, elected officials, and other organized bodies as groups, not just as individual members of the public.

In 1989, during George H.W. Bush's administration, the assistant administrator's organization was transformed into several associate administrators—one for regional, state, and local relations; one for communications and public affairs; and one for congressional and legislative affairs. Although the level was reduced from a Senate-approved appointment, we see the advent of three senior officials—two of whom specialize in the EPA's transactions with its own regional offices, other governmental partners, and Congress, and one focused on the press, stakeholders, and communities (as distinct from their elected officials). In the early 1990s, we saw the emergence for the first time of an Environmental Education division—tied to EPA intentions to be attentive to the educational aspect of its missions as well as to a law creating an Office of Environmental Education at the EPA.

In 1992 the associate administrator title was broadened to encompass communications, education, and public affairs, giving environmental education a full seat at the organizational table. This work was linked especially to engaging the education establishment and others through grants to create educational materials for various age levels.

Also in 1992, the Office of Environmental Equity was created to address specific problems outlined by both external critics and an internal task force. In 1993, during the Clinton administration, this office became the Office of Environmental Justice. In the same year the public liaison division was formed, headed by the associate administrator for communication, education, and public affairs. The Office of Environmental Justice focused on redressing the apparent disproportionate share of the burdens of environmental pollution from air and water pollution and waste disposal being borne by low-income, minority, and other disadvantaged populations. The title of the public liaison division suggested a different kind of relationship than the traditional public affairs office as well as a specific avenue for environmental, health, and consumer organizations, labor unions, industry associations, and educational and youth groups, among others, to have a clearer relationship with the agency.

In 1994 a separate and distinct Tribal Office was established to respond to the unique needs of Native American tribes, which are accorded the status of states in several EPA statutes in terms of environmental program grants and development. The office was placed within one of the agency's major program-implementation offices—the Office of Water—but was designed to serve the needs of American Indians related to all EPA programs. In 1997 the agency established an Office of Children's Health Protection, attached directly to the Office of the Administrator (U.S. EPA 1997a). Its purpose is to influence and directly impact the agency's programs that affect children.

In 1999 the Conflict Prevention and Resolution Center was established in the office of the general counsel. This center was, and continues to be, responsible for providing agency-wide advice and training on the appropriate use of alternative dispute resolution, and assistance in identifying third-party neutrals. Experience has shown that the use of techniques for preventing and resolving disputes can result in faster resolution of issues; more creative, satisfying, and enduring solutions; and increased stakeholder support for agency programs.

Although there are numerous reasons for reorganizations including mission, statutory changes, budget redirection, and even personalities, our analysis is directed at the pace and labeling of these organizational changes as it relates to engagement with members of the public, together with corresponding significant policy benchmarks. What we observe is that the tempo of such changes accelerated in the late 1980s and early 1990s as the agency sought to establish its official mechanisms for public engagement. We observe that the EPA's organizational labels for its entities that relate to individual members of the public were stable during much of the agency's early existence. Then, external relations rose in importance and the diversity of the publics needing the agency's attention grew. In addition, the creation of offices of Environmental Justice and Children's Health Protection indicate outreach and the need to engage special categories of individuals who are underrepresented by traditional stakeholder groups. The difficulty in engaging individuals from the federal level is manifest in these numerous organizational attempts to build more direct, improved connections.

We also note that the language of public affairs is grounded in a more transaction-based context (as in corporate public affairs departments). The more interactively grounded titles, such as public awareness and the concept of liaison, which the dictionary suggests is based on a close relationship rather than a transaction, imply that the EPA's organizational changes were directed at getting more closely in touch with the public.

In 1994 the Public Participation and Accountability Subcommittee of the National Environmental Justice Advisory Council, a federal advisory committee to the agency, published *The Model Plan for Public Participation*. This plan was developed as a tool for use by federal and state agencies to guide the public participation process. The model plan provided two guiding principles for public participation: (1) encourage public participation in all aspects of environmental decision making, and (2) maintain honesty and integrity in the process and articulate goals, expectations, and limitations. The model plan also outlined critical elements in successful efforts to engage public participation in environmental decision making including: (1) up-front planning to ensure agencies provide the necessary resources needed to allow the public to participate, (2) identification of diverse stakeholders, (3) recognition of the importance of making meetings accessible and open to all who wish to attend, and (4) ensuring meetings with the public have clear goals and are followed up by an action plan. The model plan also incorporated the International Association for Public Participation's "Core Values for the Practice of Public Participation" (International Association for Public Participation [IAP] 1996).

In 2003, after three years of development, internal review, and public discussion, the EPA released its Public Involvement Policy (U.S. EPA 2003b). The new policy updated the EPA's 1981 public participation policy. It recognized the changing needs of the public; introduced new statutes and regulations, new and expanded public participation techniques, and new options for public access to information including involvement through the Internet; and indicated the agency's emphasis on ensuring compliance, increased use of partnerships and technical assistance, and increased capacity of states, tribes, and local governments to carry out delegated programs (U.S. EPA 2003b).

Former EPA administrator Michael Leavitt emphasized collaborative problem solving, and under his leadership the agency developed seven keys for successful collaborations: a shared problem, a convener of stature, a committed leader, representatives of substance, a clearly defined purpose, a formal charter, and a common information base. Though there were no organizational changes, collaboration began to be considered more routinely in planning and implementation of EPA's programs. (U.S. EPA 2010a).

On April 23, 2009, Administrator Lisa Jackson issued a memorandum on "Transparency in EPA's Operations." She reaffirmed Ruckelshaus's commitment that the EPA would operate "in a fishbowl," and that the agency would provide for the fullest possible public participation in decision making by remaining open and accessible to those representing all points of view. She also directed the EPA to take affirmative steps to solicit the views of those who would be affected by agency decisions (Jackson 2009).

Statutory and Program Mandates

At the same time these shifts in the nature of the environmental protection mission and organizational and policy changes were taking place, there was an increasing demand in EPA statutes and in implementation of associated programs to perfect the agency's ability to engage the public at the individual level. The experiences we cite here are in large measure drawn from the EPA's statutes and programs on waste management; thus, they are not a random "sample" from across the EPA. They are drawn from several programs that are typically involved in site-specific actions affecting nearby residents (i.e., cleanup decisions at Superfund sites, permitting of incinerators, etc.). In contrast, most of the EPA's programs are conducted at the national level, with the agency acting as the federal regulator with delegated state programs. Thus, it is often the state government that is engaged with the public on the implementation of air and water regulation.

Several mandates from the mid-1980s were focused on improving the agency's engagement with individuals. The first was contained in the 1984 amendments to the Resource Conservation and Recovery Act, which appoint an ombudsman on waste-management issues. Here was a statutory message that the existing organizational structures were not sufficient to solve problems raised and that an advocate for resolution was needed within the organization. Although one could argue that the Office of the Ombudsman is equally available to individual companies with regulatory and compliance questions, it was still a statement of need for easier access and better engagement. Later on, the EPA established ombudsmen for waste programs in each of its ten regional offices—high-level employees who serve as points of contact for members of the public who have concerns about Superfund activities, and who can look independently into these concerns. In July 2003, the title of Superfund Regional Ombudsman was changed to Regional Public Liaison Manager (U.S. EPA 2010g).

In 1986, amendments to the Superfund law added a number of statutory requirements for public participation in the cleanup of sites on the National Priorities List. Notable among the requirements was that proposed cleanup plans had to be made available to the public for review and comment, and the agency was given the authority to award technical assistance grants (TAGs) to communities affected by the EPA's waste cleanup decisions (U.S. EPA 1992a). TAGs provide money for qualified community groups to hire independent technical advisors to interpret and help the community understand technical information about their site, and to allow their authentic engagement with the remedy decisions. The provision of technical assistance to communities continues to be an important resource and one that has more fully empowered local residents to understand and have valid input into the decision-making process that affects their immediate environment.

One of the most significant program mandates with respect to public engagement was a response to grassroots community movements rather than

134 WALTER W. KOVALICK JR., ALAN WALTS, AND SUZANNE WELLS

to statutory change. Early in 1990, the Congressional Black Caucus and a bipartisan coalition of academics, social scientists, and political activists met with EPA officials to discuss their findings. Their research indicated that environmental risk was higher for minority and low-income populations. In 1992, responding to several important critiques and reports on the issue of environmental contamination disproportionately affecting minority and low-income populations, the EPA prepared a report, "Environmental Equity: Reducing Risks for All Communities" (U.S. EPA 1992b), with a series of findings and recommendations. One finding was that these populations have higher than average exposure to certain air pollutants, hazardous waste facilities, and contaminated fish and agricultural pesticides in the workplace. The previously mentioned Office of Environmental Equity was formed at this time.

On February 11, 1994, President Bill Clinton signed Executive Order 12898, "Federal Actions to Address Environmental Justice in Minority Populations and Low-Income Populations." The order directed federal agencies to make environmental justice integral to their missions by developing environmental justice strategies to address disproportionately high and adverse human health or environmental effects of their programs on minority and low-income populations. The Presidential Memorandum accompanying the order underscored certain provisions of existing law to be applied in achieving this directive, including the nondiscrimination requirements of Title VI of the Civil Rights Act of 1964.

The executive order also established an Interagency Working Group on environmental justice chaired by the EPA administrator and comprised of the heads of eleven departments or agencies and several White House offices.[5] In 2000, the IWG group created an "Integrated Federal Interagency Environmental Justice Action Agenda" (U.S. EPA 2000), which offered an important model for public engagement in addressing environmental justice concerns. This model has continued to develop and is referred to as "collaborative problem-solving."[6] It begins to define the EPA's emerging role as an environmental steward and a "curious collaborator" (discussed later) in response to the challenges of environmental governance previously outlined.

Another development in the waste management realm was the April 1996 "Final Report of the Federal Facilities Environmental Restoration and Dialogue" Committee. Chaired by the EPA, this interagency committee conducted highly inclusive deliberations directed at the processes of stakeholder involvement in the cleanup decisions at and around federal facilities—especially those of the departments of Defense and Energy. Although primarily focused on the overall process of stakeholder interaction at these sites—many of which had been operating under a cloak of national security for decades—this discussion highlights the need to engage members of the public, including people of color and low-income individuals residing near such facilities, and their local representatives, and elaborates on how communications and, to some extent, engagement must be improved.

Outside the realm of specific waste programs, we also draw attention to two other significant initiatives that altered the EPA's institutional "styles" in engaging the public: Right to Know and Community Action for a Renewed Environment (CARE). In 1986 Congress enacted the Emergency Planning and Community Right-to-Know Act (EPCRA). EPCRA Section 313 requires the EPA and states to annually collect data on releases and transfers of certain toxic chemicals from industrial facilities and to make the data available to the public in the Toxics Release Inventory (TRI). The EPA provides these data in the "TRI Explorer," giving access to the TRI data in a form that helps communities identify facilities and chemical disposal or other release patterns that warrant further study and analysis. TRI data gives communities more information about toxic chemical management in their area and often spurs companies to focus on their chemical management practices since they are being measured and made public. From 1988 to 2008, manufacturing facilities decreased their disposal or new release of toxic substances by 65 percent. From 2007 to 2008, total disposal or other releases decreased by 257 million pounds, or 6 percent. Although this program has caused a major rearrangement of the dynamics of individual company pollution prevention and abatement programs—that is, focusing on the nature and type of unregulated releases and their volume—it has largely effected change without any EPA or state regulatory action (U.S. EPA 2010b).

Second, in 2005, the agency started the CARE program, a competitive grant program that supports community-based partnerships for projects that develop innovative, local solutions to address the risks from multiple sources of toxic pollution. This program began as a result of recommendations contained in the 2004 NEJAC report on cumulative risks and impacts (NEJAC 2004). Through CARE, various local organizations including nonprofits, businesses, schools, and governments create partnerships that implement local solutions to reduce releases of toxic pollutants and minimize people's exposure to them. The National Academy of Public Administration released a report in 2009 on the CARE program saying it has demonstrated how communities can effectively address environmental problems, and recommending ways the EPA can work with communities more effectively for mutual gain (National Academy of Public Administration 2009).

Impact of Information Technology

As we noted in the first edition of this book, all of the EPA's programs have included organized and dedicated efforts to communicate information about

136   WALTER W. KOVALICK JR., ALAN WALTS, AND SUZANNE WELLS

their direction and implementation. By that we mean long-standing efforts in the various programs to develop fact sheets, guidance, handbooks, decision maker's guides, citizen guides, newsletters, and Web pages to better outline, explain, and elaborate on regulatory requirements to numerous audiences. In many cases, these materials were also "rolled up" by the public affairs office into more generic explanatory guides and descriptive materials on the EPA's programs and regulations.

These efforts were primarily focused on outreach, information dissemination, and communication about the process of regulatory development, as well as on enhancing understanding of and compliance with regulatory requirements. With advances in information technology, and in service of its transparency goals, the EPA continues to work on improved information sharing. For example, the public can access geospatial analytical tools that provide environmental information across a range of EPA data sets and specific to their location displayed on easy-to-understand maps (U.S. EPA 2010c), as well as information on compliance status of regulated facilities (U.S. EPA 2010d). Other Web-based tools identify resources for undertaking community-based work (U.S. EPA 2010e). The EPA has also made it possible to lodge citizen complaints about potential violations of environmental law using an online form (U.S. EPA 2010f).

As the EPA builds this capacity, it also increasingly uses a range of information technologies to support dialogue and information exchange as well as outreach. Between July 2007 and Earth Day 2008, former EPA deputy administrator Marcus Peacock used a blog called "Flow of the River" to share with the public what the EPA was doing to improve its operations and make what the EPA does more open to the public. Since that first foray into blogging, Greenversations, the official blog of the EPA has been established (blog.epa.gov/blog). The EPA now accepts public comments online, and is using Facebook, Twitter, and YouTube to engage the public and encourage online information sharing.

Evolution of Roles

We believe that subsequent developments affirm the role of the public administrator as a "task-oriented, but inclusive and balanced convener," as set out in the first edition of this book. However, that role is continuing to evolve and to be given more specific content as the EPA more routinely employs approaches such as collaborative problem solving and the governance model of environmental stewardship to address challenges that cannot be met through single or multiple regulatory interventions alone. We describe this emerging role—the next horizon in the EPA's ongoing evolution—as that of a curious collaborator.

The study "Public Knowledge and Perceptions of Chemical Risks in Six Communities: Analysis of a Baseline Survey" (U.S. EPA 1991) is very instructive on the difficulty for government in establishing effective interaction with individuals. When more than 3,000 persons were surveyed on a variety of questions related to chemical risks, they were asked where they received most of their information, whom they trusted for this information, and whom they thought was most knowledgeable about these risks. Regarding the source for their information, news reporters and environmental groups were chosen by 27 percent and 21 percent of the respondents, respectively. Local, state, and federal government ranked at 5 percent or below. On the issue of whom they most trusted, doctors were chosen by 46 percent, with governments ranking at 12 percent or below and the chemical industry at 8 percent. Lastly, as to who is most knowledgeable, the respondents named chemical industry officials (58 percent), followed by environmental groups (53 percent) and the federal government (36 percent).

At a minimum, one sees in these data no congruence in information sources, authoritative voices, or technical information providers. In addition, the low ranking of governments in general and the federal government in particular, except for its scientific assets, gives credence to the kind of role we see evolving.

Although our portrait of developments in the complexity of environmental protection, the EPA's organizational evolution, and programmatic change is abbreviated and incomplete, we think it conveys a sense of development and transition in the roles played by the EPA in carrying out its mission with and through individuals. We suggest that there are at least four major roles that the agency has played in its evolutionary engagement with individuals.

The first role was that of the *authority,* which the *American Heritage College Dictionary* (Third edition 1993) describes as "an *accepted* source of expert information or advice; power to influence or persuade resulting from knowledge or experience" [italics added]. In exercising its discretion to interpret statutes and write regulations, the EPA was the preeminent authority on solving what were the more obvious and visible problems of the 1970s. Its engagement with the outside world—let alone individual members of the public—was the dissemination of information about its actions, the reasons behind them, and the results. In these times, there were no disagreements about the nature of the problems (i.e., the many large industrial sources of pollution), let alone the apparent solutions. So the EPA was the trusted purveyor of the "facts and figures" about the problems of the environment and what needed to be done about them. There was less need for individuals to be engaged in decision making as the agency was new, making progress on obvious fronts, and appeared to be exercising its discretion on behalf of the public interest.

The second role was that of *neutral arbiter*. An agency anecdote in the late 1970s and 1980s was that if the EPA issued a regulation and was immediately sued by both industry and the environmentalists (i.e., national environmental organizations), the EPA must have "gotten it about right." Gone were the days of the trusted public agent. The agency was responsible for making a regulatory proposal, hearing from all sides, and, based on that input (and presumably its expertise), making the decision that met its statutory responsibility to protect public health and the environment. This was a time of increasing complexity of problems with less obvious solutions.

The EPA sought heightened public awareness (rather than pure information dissemination) and tried to move beyond the organized interest groups to include the public at large. But as we saw organizationally, the collected publics became further and further differentiated into states, tribes, cities, elected officials, and industry, with the individual members of the public not obvious on the regulatory scene. Late in this period came the realization about environmental education—that giving students, their parents, and communities a background in environmental issues promises more environmentally conscious adults now and in the future. Thus, the agency was no longer perceived as principal information purveyor, but began to empower others to learn about these issues and to call on the broader science community for information. Then, and now, the call for "good science" began to be heard in order to still debates on regulatory decisions that lacked sufficient anchors in the "truth."

In the meantime, immediate fixes were sought through laws requiring an ombudsman and providing grant funds to allow community members around Superfund sites to choose their own technical advisors on complicated scientific and technical issues. Community involvement became the watchword for developing solutions at Superfund sites, even though the EPA was still making the decisions about remedies at these sites.

During the 1990s, the EPA evolved in its regulatory, voluntary, and partnership efforts, and, even in its site-specific work, as the task-oriented, but inclusive and balanced convener. The agency retains its statutory responsibility to exercise discretion in the interest of public health and the environment, and it still has its technical and scientific assets to draw on. However, many of its nonregulatory programs that were established at this time dealt with problems for which the agency's technical expertise is not unique or comprehensive—especially given the diverse and widespread problems faced by its traditional programs (nonpoint source pollution in water [e.g., agricultural and urban runoff], thousands of leaking underground tanks, and so on). In addition, the answers to complex scientific and risk assessment questions come from numerous sources—some trusted even more than the EPA. So it follows that the EPA became the *convener*—"one who causes people to assemble, usually for an official or public purpose" (*American Heritage College Dictionary,* 1993). The agency is being trusted to bring all the interests to the table and to be balanced in moderating the debate on the question at hand. In addition, in matters of regulation, the EPA is still driven by its statutory mandates to protect public health and the environment, so its role is beyond the neutral facilitator. It is the explicit final decision maker in regulatory programs, less so in voluntary programs. But in either case, the agency has an agenda for completion of the project or achievement of the goal—often statutorily driven. Hence, the concept of task orientation, which is the need to keep the process moving to conclusion, to exercise governance over the "group process," and to persuade and, if necessary, overrule those who would hold veto power in what might be a consensus process.

It is in this role that the EPA found itself moving beyond information transmission to members of the public and beyond being the judge of submitted views (especially when public views were not articulated). The EPA must be trusted to ensure that all views are represented in the decision-making process—especially of those who need help in understanding the technical issues—to make sure no one is drowned out or is too timid to speak, to use its own scientific and technical assets, and to operate a transparent decision process for all concerned. So we add to the role of convener the responsibilities of task orientation as well as inclusiveness and balanced treatment. The distance from the authoritative role is great, and the journey was not direct, but the resulting engagement moves ever closer to connecting directly to the needs of individuals.

Now we see the EPA moving to occupy a new role—that of a curious collaborator. Curiosity means, in this context, the commitment to authentic efforts to learn through dialogue not only what problems are to be solved, but also what the EPA's role is in achieving solutions. The EPA increasingly employs inquiry as much as advocacy to discover the best means to create needed change in the face of systemic issues—where no single authority or expert can ensure an optimal outcome (or even define what is optimal). This is in fact the situation in which we have always found ourselves, but the agency faces it more directly today as the complexity of the problems is more and more matched only by the urgency of resolving them, and as the sophistication and capacity of the affected public to offer views grows exponentially in concert with information technology. These technologies enable members of the public to organize as groups and to identify needs and solutions (often using information collected and disseminated by the EPA and other regulatory agencies).

The EPA has a long history of efforts to adapt and modify the existing

140 WALTER W. KOVALICK JR., ALAN WALTS, AND SUZANNE WELLS

regulatory regimes originally designed to address specific media (e.g., air, water, land) to better function at an ecosystem and community scale.[7] This chapter focuses on certain examples of that adaptation in terms of how the EPA interacts with individuals who are members of communities and civic organizations. Solutions to environmental problems must embrace ecosystem and community scales, rather than solely operating in terms of (industrial) sectors and media. Responding to such problems requires different approaches to governance that are founded on shared stewardship norms in addition to regulatory norms.

Norms are defined here as shared assumptions (implicit or explicit theories) about how to *appropriately* and *effectively* take collective action. These shared assumptions determine what problems ought to be solved and identify causes of those problems. They also establish the collective means through which norms will be enacted, enforced, and modified in response to changing circumstances. *Governance* can then be defined as how society steers itself by these collective means (the word *govern* derives from the Latin *gubernare,* "to steer, govern").

Regulatory norms are enacted as rules that command certain actions and control behavior. They are enforced by a governing organization with the authority to require compliance. Means of imposing compliance include punishing to deter future violations, restoring equity by recovering the economic benefit of violations, and restoring full compliance by requiring remedial action. The effectiveness of these norms in protecting the public and the environment from harm depends on (a) how effectively and efficiently their regulatory purpose is met and (b) how effectively and efficiently the regulators ensure compliance with them. However, as discussed earlier, regulatory norms are best suited to enable vigorous and direct response to highly significant and relatively isolable challenges, such as concentrated streams of effluent and emissions from specific locations. Given such challenges, regulatory responses focus on effected media (air, water, land) and on significant localized impacts (stationary sources, point sources), and apply emissions standards or technology-based standards by media and facility.

However, many of the most salient and urgent problems now present themselves in terms of pervasive, multiple, and cumulative challenges, such as climate change, nonpoint source water pollution, and many environmental justice issues. In addition, work at an ecosystem and community scale inherently focuses attention on the overall health or sustainability of these systems and on the interdependence of the actors within those systems. Stewardship norms are codes of conduct that define some actions and outcomes as desirable on sustainability grounds and others as undesirable, whether or not those actions and outcomes are amenable to command and control. They

THE EPA SEEKS ITS ROLE IN COMMUNITIES   141

are enforced through governing mechanisms that are jointly owned by those with recognized interests, and that enforcement depends on the transparent exchange of accurate information on a basis of joint accountability rather than on unilateral control.

The agency necessarily acts in terms of both stewardship norms and regulatory norms. However, as stewardship norms become more critical—as the environmental challenges become more complicated and less amenable to "command and control" regulation; or, alternatively, as success with command and control regulation and increased analytical capacity creates opportunities to address systemic challenges—regulators must consider these norms more explicitly. They must also seek forms of governance that can more effectively coordinate how existing programs are being administered; and more effectively enable collaboration in problem-solving efforts.

This is clearly an immense and ongoing challenge, but one that calls for incremental changes with the growth of our scientific capacity to evaluate and our civic capacity to act. In addition, these changes have evolved; stewardship does not replace regulation. In terms of community involvement, the various roles that the EPA has occupied over the years are not mutually exclusive, when viewed in light of different levels for stakeholder interaction that guide most public environmental decision-making efforts. The International Association for Public Participation's model of this "Spectrum of Participation" ranges (in order of increasing public impact on the outcome) from outreach, to information exchange, to seeking recommendation, to reaching agreements, to empowering stakeholders to take action (IAP 2007). There are many specific circumstances in which the EPA should provide information (as an authority or expert) or obtain advice or comments (as a decision maker or arbiter). However, as the challenges of environmental, economic, and social sustainability become more central to the EPA's work, it increasingly must collaborate and empower as well. This evolving role is graphically presented in Figure 8.1, developed to show the different collaborative approaches the EPA uses depending on the issue and desired outcome of the stakeholder interaction process.

Along with the logic of the EPA's public participation policies and training, there is significant evidence of this direction in recent developments. A recent report from an outside advisory committee states that the EPA should "reframe its mission with stewardship as the unifying theme and ethic," and notes that the EPA can realize an ethic of stewardship only through collaboration (National Advisory Committee on Environmental Policy and Technology 2008). The implications extend well beyond the scope of this chapter, as evident from the definition given for stewardship: "a systemic approach to addressing the challenge of sustainability—economic, environmental, and social" (U.S. EPA

Figure 8.1 **Public Involvement Spectrum: A Range Possible of Processes**

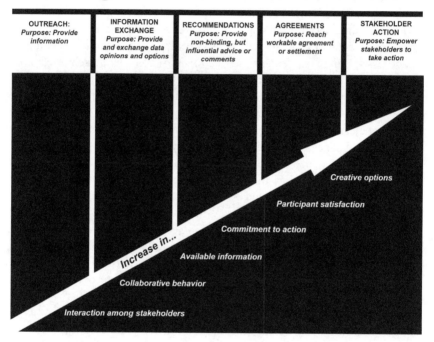

2008). This approach argues for strong regulatory programs as well as a suite of other approaches to achieving sustainability. With respect to public involvement in particular, however, it calls on the EPA to "foster stewardship by providing leadership in collaborative governance and participating in partnerships organized by others" (U.S. EPA 2008). As noted earlier, NACEPT has been charged with building on these recommendations and is helping the EPA to determine how to integrate these stewardship principles further into its work.

More evidence is found in the approach being tested in the environmental justice context (and others) through the collaborative problem-solving model. The EPA's environmental justice program continues its efforts to institutionalize this model as one way in which the EPA can empower communities and individuals. The EPA has also undertaken a range of other efforts to build civic capacity, such as by developing tools and providing funding to groups that work on issues at a watershed (or other place-based) level (Sirianni 2009).

The Evolving Relationship between the EPA and the Public

Notable among federal agencies, the EPA's purview and statutes require it to be engaged at the "retail" level with members of the public relating to the air they breathe, the water they drink, the risks associated with their homes in proximity to industrial and waste sites, the safety of food treated with pesticides, the expected mileage from their new car, and the list goes on. As the agency enters its fortieth year, we argue that many statutory and policy underpinnings and social and technological developments have helped shape the framework for public engagement and involvement in the agency's work to protect public health and the environment. We clearly recognize the bulk of this public engagement is conducted with and through partners in state, local, and tribal governments, since the vast majority of implementation (e.g., permits, inspections, enforcement actions, and so on) takes place at those levels. Nonetheless, EPA staff often end up at the front lines as spokespeople for agency action on these many issues. In our view, the hallmark for the EPA's practice and the models discussed here is their evolutionary nature in terms of adapting to both legislative and public policy outcomes as well as to changes in public awareness of broader environmental issues, increased "professionalism" of public engagement due to networking, advances in information technology, and other societal influences.

In 2010 there appears to be a deeper understanding that authentic engagement with the public enhances the quality of government decisions. President Obama and EPA administrator Lisa Jackson have expressed their commitment to uphold the values of transparency and openness in conducting government operations. Administrator Jackson issued her "Transparency in EPA Operations" memo in April 2009, which committed the agency to "provide for the fullest possible public participation in decision making." As environmental problems become more pervasive and urgent, as the concepts of sustainability and environmental stewardship continue to morph and evolve in society, and as the public demands a greater role in environmental decision making, the EPA also will have to adapt and move beyond the concepts we have suggested in this chapter.

Notes

The opinions expressed in this chapter are those of the authors and do not necessarily represent the views of the United States Environmental Protection Agency.

1. See, for example, the Pew Internet and American Life Project report on "The Internet and Civic Engagement" (Sept. 2009), http://www.pewinternet.org/Reports/2009/15--The-Internet-and-Civic-Engagement.aspx, accessed January 2010.

144 WALTER W. KOVALICK JR., ALAN WALTS, AND SUZANNE WELLS

2. Administrator Lisa Jackson has established a NACEPT subcommittee on promoting environmental stewardship that "will provide advice on how to promote environmental stewardship practices that encompass all environmental aspects of an organization in the regulated community and other sectors, as appropriate, in order to enhance environmental protection and human health." (Letter from Administrator Jackson to Erik Meyers, July 7, 2009, http://www.epa.gov/ocem/nacept/reports/pdf/2009_07_nacept_oultook_for_epa_response.pdf, retrieved January 19, 2011.)

3. Oral history interview of William D. Ruckelshaus, available at http://earth1.epa.gov/history/publications/ruck/14.htm, accessed January 2010.

4. See http://www.epa.gov/region9/kettleman/, accessed January 2010. This site provides documents including the draft EJ assessment, which summarizes responses to comments including requiring the permit applicant to conduct additional sampling.

5. These include the EPA, the departments of Justice, Defense, Energy, Labor, Interior, Transportation, Agriculture, Housing and Urban Development, Commerce, and Health and Human Services, as well as the Council on Environmental Quality, the Office of Management and Budget, the Office of Science and Technology Policy, the Domestic Policy Council, and the Council of Economic Advisors.

6. See http://www.epa.gov/compliance/ej/resources/publications/grants/cps-manual-12-27-06.pdf, accessed January 19, 2011. Several case studies of collaborative problem solving to address environmental justice concerns are found in "Models for Success" (EPA-300-R-08-005, August 2008) and "EPA's EJ Collaborative Problem-Solving Model" (EPA-300-R-06-002, June 2008).

7. The EPA's efforts to collaboratively govern at a watershed scale, as well as the challenges it faces in doing so, are discussed in Sirianni (2009). The EPA's Community Action for a Renewed Environment (CARE) Resource Guide collects EPA resources that support community-based work; available at http://www.epa.gov/care/library/howto.pdf, accessed January 2010.

References

American Heritage College Dictionary, 3d ed. 1993. Boston: Houghton Mifflin Co.
Environmental Justice Resource Center. Undated. "Shintech Throws in Towel on Environmental Racism Case." Available at http://www.ejrc.cau.edu/shintechvic.html, accessed January 19, 2011.
Hallissy, Erin. 1997. "Unocal Will Settle Suits for $80 Million." *San Francisco Chronicle,* April 15, A1.
International Association of Public Participation. 2007. "IAP2 Spectrum of Public Participation." Available at www.iap2.0rg/associations/4748/files/IAP2%20 Spectrum_vertical.pdf, accessed January 2010.
———. 1996. "Core Values for the Practice of Public Participation." Available at http://iap2.affiniscape.com/associations/4748/files/CoreValues.pdf, accessed January 2010.
Jackson, Lisa. 2009. "Memo to EPA Employees: Transparency in EPA's Operations," April 23. Available at http://www.epa.gov/Administrator/operationsmemo.html, accessed November 22, 2010.
Kuehn, Robert. 1996. "Environmental Justice Implications of Quantitative Risk Assessment." *University of Illinois Law Review* 103 (38): 103–72.
Louisiana Environmental Action Network. 2004. Demographic Data Report, April 7. Available at http://data.leanweb.org/news/lean_217.html, accessed January 19, 2011.

Medina-Vera, Myriam, J.M. Van Emon, L.J. Melnyk, K.D. Bradham, S.L. Harper, and J.N. Morgan. 2010. "An Overview of Measurement Method Tools Available to Communities for Conducting Exposure and Cumulative Risk Assessments." *Journal of Exposure Science and Environmental Epidemiology* 20 (4): 1–12.

National Academy of Public Administration. 2009. "Putting Community First: A Promising Approach to Federal Collaboration for Environmental Improvement." Washington, DC: NAPA.

National Advisory Committee on Environmental Policy and Technology. 2008. "Everyone's Business: Working towards Sustainability through Environmental Stewardship and Collaboration." Washington, DC: Environmental Protection Agency.

National Environmental Justice Advisory Council (NEJAC). 2004. "Ensuring Risk Reduction in Communities with Multiple Stressors: Environmental Justice and Cumulative Risks/Impacts." Cumulative Risks/Impacts Work Group Report, December. Washington, DC: Environmental Protection Agency.

National Research Council. 1983. *Risk Assessment in the Federal Government: Managing the Process.* Washington, DC: National Academy Press.

———. 1994. *Science and Judgment in Risk Assessment.* Washington, DC: National Academy Press.

Sirianni, Carmen. 2009. "The Civic Mission of a Federal Agency in the Age of Networked Governance." *American Behavioral Scientist* 52 (6): 933, 939.

U.S. Environmental Protection Agency (EPA). 1970. Reorganization Plan No. 3 of 1970. Special Message from the President to the Congress about Reorganization Plans to Establish the Environmental Protection Agency and the National Oceanic and Atmospheric Administration, July 9. Available at http://www.epa.gov/history/org/origins/reorg.htm, accessed January 2010.

———. 1990. "Reducing Risk, Setting Priorities and Strategies for Environmental Protection." Washington, DC.

———. 1991. "Public Knowledge and Perceptions of Chemical Risks in Six Communities: Analysis of a Baseline Survey." Washington, DC: Chemical Emergency Planning and Preparedness Office.

———. 1992a. "CERCLA/Superfund Orientation Manual." Washington, DC: Office of Solid Waste and Emergency Response.

———. 1992b. "Environmental Equity: Reducing Risks for All Communities." Washington, D.C: Office of Policy, Planning, and Evaluation.

———. 1993. "Oral History Interview: William D. Ruckelshaus." Available at http://www.epa.gov/history/publications/print/ruck.htm, accessed November 22, 2010.

———. 1997a. "Community-Based Environmental Protection: A Resource Book for Protecting Ecoysystems and Communities." Washington, DC: Offfice of Policy, Planning, and Evaluation.

———. 1997b. Science Policy Council. Guidance on Cumulative Risk Assessment, Part 1: Planning and Scoping. Office of the Science Advisor. Available at http://www.epa.gov/OSA/spc/2cumrisk.htm, accessed November 22, 2010.

———. 2000. "Integrated Federal Interagency Environmental Justice Action Agenda." Available at http://www.epa.gov/compliance/ej/resources/publications/interagency/actionagenda.pdf, accessed January 20, 2011.

———. 2003a. "Framework for Cumulative Risk Assessment." Office of Research and Development, National Center for Environmental Assessment. Available at http://oaspub.epa.gov/eims/eimscomm.getfile?p_download_id=36941, accessed January 20, 2011.

———. 2003b. "Public Involvement Policy of the U.S. Environmental Protection Agency." Office of Policy, Economics and Innovation. Available at http://www.epa.gov/publicinvolvement/policy2003/index.htm, accessed November 22, 2010.

———. 2007. "Concepts, Methods and Data Sources for Cumulative Health Risk Assessment of Multiple Chemicals, Exposures and Effects." Cincinnati, OH: Office of Research and Development, National Center for Environmental Assessment.

———. 2008. "Working Together: An Introduction to Collaborative Decision Making." Washington, DC.

———. 2010a. "Collaborative Problem-Solving." Office of Strategic Environmental Management. Available at http://www.epa.gov/publicinvolvement/collaboration/, accessed November 22, 2010.

———. 2010b. "What Is the Toxics Release Inventory Program?" Toxics Release Inventory Program. Available at http://www.epa.gov/TRI/triprogram/whatis.htm, accessed November 22, 2010.

———. 2010c. "My Environment." Available at www.epa.gov/myenvironment/, accessed November 22, 2010.

———. 2010d. U.S. EPA. 2010d. "Enforcement and Compliance History Online (ECHO)." Compliance and Enforcement Home. Available at www.epa.gov/compliance/data/systems/multimedia/echo.html, accessed January 2010.

———. 2010e. "Community Action for a Renewed Environment (CARE)." CARE. Available at http://www.epa.gov/air/care/index.htm, accessed January 1, 2010.

———. 2010f. "Compliance and Enforcement." Available at http://www.epa.gov/compliance/complaints/index.html, accessed January 1, 2010.

———. 2010g. Regional Public Liaison Program, Office of Superfund Remediation and Technology Innovation. Available at http://www.epa.gov/superfund/community/rpl, accessed October 1, 2010.

U.S. Government. 1981. "Responsiveness Summary and Preamble on Public Participation, Final E.P.A. Policy on Public Participation" 46 Federal Register 12 (19 January 1981), 5736–746.

U.S. Government General Accounting Office. 1994. "Issues Pertaining to an Incinerator in East Liverpool, Ohio." Washington, DC: Author.

U.S. Office of Management and Budget. 1996. "Economic Analysis of Federal Regulation under Executive Order 12866." Whitehouse.gov, January 11. Available at http://www.whitehouse.gov/omb/inforeg_riaguide, accessed November 22, 2010.

U.S. Supreme Court. 2009. *Entergy Corp. v. Riverkeeper, Inc.* Available at http://www.supremecourt.gov/opinions/08pdf/07–588.pdf, accessed November 22, 2010.

Yamashita, Eiji. 2009. "Feds Host Meeting on PCB Plan for Kettleman." *Hanford Sentinel,* February 5.

Zartarian, Valerie, and Bradley D. Schultz. 2009. "The EPA's Human Exposure Research Program for Assessing Cumulative Risk in Communities." *Journal of Exposure Science and Environmental Epidemiology* 20 4: 1–8.1.

9

Obituary

Team Metro

Claire Mostel

Residents of unincorporated Miami-Dade County are mourning the death of Team Metro. The county department that put a face on local government passed away on September 30, 2008. It is survived by loyal staff members and county residents who appreciated having a government office in their neighborhood.

Residents loved having a county office in a convenient location that provided a variety of government outreach services, including the ability to apply for a U.S. passport or purchase Metrorail passes or tokens, and dog licenses Of course, those residents that received the punitive side (code violations/civil citations) of Team Metro were not as happy with the department. But everyone agrees on one thing: they will miss having Team Metro in their neighborhood.

Residents seeking the services formerly provided by Team Metro can contact the Office of Neighborhood Compliance (ONC) or the Government Information Center (GIC). In lieu of flowers or donations, citizens are asked to continue to participate in their local government and hold it accountable to its residents.

After a glorious fourteen-year run of providing excellent customer service, the cause of death is rumored to be politics and budget cuts. An autopsy will be conducted to determine the actual cause; the results of the investigation and thoughts on what, if anything, could have been done to prevent this sad event will follow.

In the Beginning

Team Metro was born in a trailer after Hurricane Andrew blew through the South Dade section of Miami-Dade County. From devastation grew a concept of bringing government closer to its citizens, especially in times of crisis . . . a new day in local government!

148   CLAIRE MOSTEL

On August 24, 1992, Dade County residents got ready for a hurricane; no one had an inkling of the magnitude of damage Hurricane Andrew would dump on South Dade County. Andrew would change the lives of many, including myself. Little did I know that three years later its impact would change my career path and my life.

Although I was already working in the public sector in 1992, I didn't realize how little I really knew about government until June 12, 1995. That was the day I started working for Team Metro.

Hurricane Andrew was supposed to hit somewhere between downtown Miami and southern Broward County (north of Miami-Dade County). However, Andrew had a mind of his own, as most storms do, and instead whirled its way through South Dade, about twenty miles south of the county government seat. At that time, the region was a largely agricultural area not as densely populated as the rest of the county. In the wake of Andrew, County Manager Joaquin Avino decided to put a trailer next to the ravaged South Dade Government Center to house county staff; this gave the residents of the South Dade area access to government services to start rebuilding their destroyed homes and lives. This unit was called Project CHART (Coordinated Hurricane Andrew Response Team)—the person charged with running the operation was Debbie Curtin.

In the fall of 1994, the manager decided that Project CHART was so successful at bringing government services closer to those who needed them, that he created Team Metro. The concept was to create regional offices throughout unincorporated Miami-Dade County that would act as mini city halls. The original Project CHART office turned into the Team Metro South Dade Office, and eight additional offices followed, as well as the administrative office located downtown in the real county hall. What started out as an information and referral service quickly blossomed into community outreach—it was a very exciting time. We were immersed in training, attending meetings and events, and, in the process, became the face of the county. If you didn't know who to contact to resolve a problem, you'd call Team Metro. Things taking too long to be resolved? Call Team Metro. Don't know what government services are available? Team Metro knew and was only too happy to come to your meeting and tell you.

A typical day usually involved giving information on how to access a county service or taking complaints for other county departments and referring them to the responsible parties. Our offices were information clearinghouses—a mini resource library with pamphlets and brochures containing county, state, and federal information. In the South Office, a great deal of time was spent assisting residents with problems stemming from Hurricane Andrew. We saw the good and bad of people—strangers still willing to help others and those who were still looking to capitalize on the misfortunes of others. The latter scam artists came with promises of putting homes back together, then fled with the money.

It was a wonderful time for a government junkie and child of the sixties. There was a great deal of citizen interaction: we actually helped people and saw the results of government working with and for its constituents. And citizens flexed their muscles and got the government to respond. All of these were new experiences for many. The Team Metro staff was a truly diverse group of many ethnicities, races, genders, ages, and sexual orientations. We came from diverse professional backgrounds (many different county departments), but we all had one thing in common: a strong commitment to improving the quality of life in Miami-Dade County. We were also free spirits, a trait embraced by our director. She encouraged us to take local government services in a new direction, creating new opportunities and building relationships with residents, community groups, civic organizations, and the business community. We also established relationships with county commissioners, assisting or partnering with them on community projects. Team Metro was everywhere, doing everything.

Our department was small. We started with just forty-seven people. Close personal relationships were fostered by numerous night meetings and weekend events. That closeness was cemented by our common interests in helping people and serving the community, and the idea that we were an "elite" department. The benefits from such cohesiveness included information sharing, resource sharing, covering for each other, and working together on different projects throughout our large county.

Team Metro was originally part of the county manager's office. In October 1995, it became a free-standing department. As a result of Debbie Curtin's vision and the success of the organization, it was apparent that Team Metro had the capacity to be more than an information source and referral machine. By January 1996, the department began to absorb areas of code enforcement from the public works, zoning, and solid waste departments. The solid waste experiment didn't last long, and that function eventually went back home. But the other enforcement functions—all quality-of-life areas—remained. Now we were able to control our own destiny. There was no need to chase after other departments for code enforcement issues because our staff took care of that. Outreach was also expanding. Team Metro created, implemented, or partnered in all major events taking place in the county, including beautification projects for residents and schools. We became adept at squeezing donations of goods and money from businesses for projects and became experts on butterfly gardens. We were everywhere!

Once code enforcement became one of Team Metro's responsibilities,

150   CLAIRE MOSTEL

Box 9.1

"I have come to look forward to each of the meetings and especially looking forward to what I was going to learn. I definitely feel more empowered. I truly feel that if I come to a problem I have my trusty black spiral notebook (minus a few numbers); knowing full well that somewhere in that notebook will be a solution to my problem."

—T. Maxwell

---

the department became schizophrenic—a helping hand on the outreach side and a hammer on the code enforcement side. This problem with our identity contributed to our demise—who were we? How could we go to night meetings and deal with citizens' concerns and the next morning give those same citizens code enforcement citations? It was quite a balancing act and at times gave us many headaches.

In a continued quest to bring services closer to residents, we started moving in another direction. In 1996, Team Metro became an authorized U.S. passport agent. This became a profitable enterprise but later contributed to our downfall. We also sold transit passes, baby stroller parking permits, and dog licenses. We gave tests for bike-and-ride passes. Our offices served as the distribution point for any new program that was being rolled out. When the housing department opened its Section 8 applications list, our offices had long lines of people waiting outside to register. Residents loved the ease of going to their local Team Metro office for one-stop government services.

In addition to code enforcement and direct sales, outreach was stretching to new areas. Initially staff took part in various existing community events and projects. But later, staff members began to create them: graffiti paint-outs, litter pick-ups, beautification projects, butterfly gardens, and education programs to name a few. After a hurricane, our staff delivered ice and water, and became agents for the Federal Emergency Management Agency's Operation Blue Roof, a program that installs plastic sheeting on homes with roof damage. Our outreach efforts also became an extension of the county commissioners' offices. When the commissioners needed help delivering turkeys or distributing book bags at back-to-school events, they called Team Metro. The list went on and on. Outreach moved outside of our realm as we started dabbling in social services. We went wherever necessary to help resolve a problem, which involved creating partnerships with other county departments, local agencies, religious organizations, schools, nonprofits, regulatory agencies, and so forth. Team Metro, the government institution, was morphing into governance.

Box 9.2

"As a Citizens' Academy graduate I know first-hand the desire that participants have to learn what department does what. I know that having completed Citizens' Academy has proved helpful to me as a county employee now."

—J. Gomez

"I have been with the county a little over a year. I just completed the most recent Team Metro Citizens' Academy at the Hammocks Library. I enrolled in this program to increase my knowledge about what different county departments do on a daily basis. My customer service skills will also benefit because I can better handle inquiries from Miami-Dade County's residents that may not pertain to my specific department. Of course, I also benefited from this program as a resident of Miami-Dade County which this program is primarily targeted for. My knowledge base on county departments and services has increased tremendously as a county resident and county employee."

—R. Valdes

Previously, local government had made decisions behind county doors and directed the delivery and direction of services. During the Team Metro period, efforts were made to include civic, business, and homeowner groups in the decision-making process. Collaboration was taking place between Team Metro and formal and informal groups representing various sectors of the county. The department created two signature programs: Neighborhood PRIDE (Partnership, Responsibility, Duty, and Enforcement) and the Citizens' Academy. Both programs had the same goals of involving residents in their communities and strengthening the bond between the community and local government. But each program took a different path to reach those goals. Both programs won National Association of Counties (NACo) Achievement Awards, were instrumental in improving community involvement and interaction, and were part of the shift from government into governance.

As the creator and coordinator of the Citizens' Academy, I had to balance providing resources and information regarding county services while maintaining transparency in how the county operated. The purpose of the academy was to transform citizen interaction with county employees, while at the same time gaining knowledge to access their local government and be able

152   CLAIRE MOSTEL

to hold that government accountable. More important, it was about building relationships among county staff members, as well as with and between the Citizens' Academy students and to encourage citizen participation and civic engagement. County residents benefited from the academy's classes. They learned how their local government operates, received hard copy information about services and contacts, and got a better picture of how their tax dollars were spent.

County employees also took part in the Citizens' Academy. It gave them the opportunity to learn about the function and operations of other departments and provided professional networking. The result was more knowledgeable county employees with increased resources.

Neighborhood PRIDE was designed to involve residents in maintaining and improving their neighborhoods while complying with code enforcement. The program started out with staff members working with residents in various parts of the county on neighborhood improvements, such as tree planting, beautification projects, and renovating properties of elderly and/ or indigent residents. However, in the last few years, a lot of the activities became festive events with inflatable bounce houses and face painting, and the focus was lost.

Each Team Metro office established a volunteer pool of people and organizations that would provide food, supplies, and money for community projects. Students who needed community hours assisted in our offices and on community projects; community hours were also available for white-collar criminals and participants in other court-ordered programs. As we progressed, the projects became more extravagant.

For all the good things the department did, Team Metro started accumulating detractors. We also lost the "protection" of our very supportive county manager, Merrett Stierheim, who became a victim of politics. After Team Metro's original department director, Debbie Curtin, retired due to illness, we seemed to lose focus and direction. Debbie provided leadership and a human touch. We wanted to do well for her; she had stood up for us when we were attacked by disgruntled citizens and county officials. She made a point of regularly visiting all Team Metro offices, not just to observe operations, but to interact with staff. Debbie encouraged input and personal growth, and made each individual feel important to the team.

Then suddenly, Team Metro was vulnerable. Due to a combination of politics and funding, we started playing the "numbers" game. The county's shift to performance management was tied into the budget, and staff members were given monthly "goals" that resulted in a shift from tangible community service to "how many?" Emphasis was no longer on quality, high-impact community events and projects. It was on quantity: how many events and

OBITUARY: TEAM METRO   153

Box 9.3

"That is a major loss to our community, that you aren't doing the program . . . thanks for the info. . . ."

—Martha

---

how extravagant. We were doing health fairs, reading to kids in schools, celebrating Grandparents' Day. These are all worthwhile activities, but we were straying from our mission.

Team Metro was no longer the fair-haired child; our golden time had passed. The communities' needs were no longer a consideration. We fought off elimination at the end of the 2006–07 fiscal year, but lacked county commission support at the end of 2007–08. The county manager and strong mayor convinced the county commissioners that the county did not need the Team Metro regional offices, and the deal-making began. After fourteen years as a neighborhood resource it was time to go. The decentralized county department was eliminated, and in its place was a centralized code enforcement department with a fraction of the outreach staff. The purpose of outreach staff had changed. The focus was no longer on being the bridge between citizens and local government. Instead, the outreach staff's purpose was to provide code enforcement education to promote voluntary compliance. The concept of having regional offices to serve communities was thrown out the window in favor of having one centralized office in a county that covers 2,000 square miles.

The Citizens' Academy was a casualty of so-called realignment. I was contacted by former students when they heard of the demise of the program. Staff from other county departments wanted to continue the program, but the resources were not available.

Team Metro's staff had eventually grown to about 250. The new department, the Office of Neighborhood Compliance, was decimated to a staff of 138. Though many have gone, many of us remain. We still carry out our mission, but with a different focus—code compliance. For most of us, in our hearts we are still Team Metro. The transition from focusing on community issues to providing code enforcement education has been difficult. It has also been a problem for county commission staff, who were used to calling Team Metro for assistance in carrying out many of their projects. It has been frustrating explaining to constituents that we no longer provide many of the services they were accustomed to receiving from Team Metro, especially since they are dealing with many of the same people. Even though staff members

154   CLAIRE MOSTEL

Box 9.4

"I am so glad that at least a small fraction of Team Metro managed to survive and you still have a job! I was flabbergasted when I heard that Team Metro was being eliminated. Your office did such a phenomenal job. Leave it to the politicians to eliminate the offices that actually benefit the public."

—M.E. Sardinas

---

follow directives to meet their new mission, it appears that there is a lack of transparency when interacting with residents.

Community reaction to the loss of Team Metro was too little too late. We received calls from homeowners' groups lamenting their loss of a one-stop government center in their community. Interestingly, staff members from other county departments were also disappointed, because they had come to rely on Team Metro as a partner and information source.

What Went Wrong?

A number of things led to the downfall of Team Metro. The most prominent included the following:

- Politics: pressure from county officials to void citations for code violations given to family, friends, and politic campaign contributors
- Politics: a department director who wasn't part of "the club"
- Incorporation movement: the need for local government to be closer to its people
- Declining proprietary revenue
- Elimination of immediate citations
- Increased rate of voluntary compliance
- Budget: available funding decreased due to shrinking property taxes

In retrospect, we also made mistakes. Unfortunately, just providing excellent public service is not enough. In order to survive, you must cultivate relationships with community members, business owners, and politicians. Each group must see the value you provide, the positive impact, and how they would be negatively affected if you were gone. While this may not be an idealistic way to look at things, it is realistic one. I am convinced that in order to survive in the jungle of government, you must be able to play the game. Not that you should sacrifice your values and ethics, but be aware of the terrain and the minefields. I don't think Team Metro/ONC ever did that.

We sat back too much, thinking that we were providing much-needed services to the community and that would be enough. But we were wrong! When all was said and done, Team Metro had no visible community support because the county's budget information was deceiving. There was very little community support before the final budget hearing. The screaming came afterwards, when it was too late. Even the county commissioners were clueless. They went along with the elimination because they each thought that *their* Team Metro office would be spared from the knife.

The handwriting was on the wall before 2008; we just weren't listening. Even now, after seeing the elimination of Team Metro and being aware of the economic environment, my staff has been slow to shift into high gear and show our value to the community. They have remained in a reactive mode, and we are now once again paying the price, although it's possible that nothing could have stopped the move to complete the process.

Citizens and county commissioners are starting to wake up and see what is happening with local government. They are realizing something is wrong with a large bureaucracy that is top heavy with highly paid attorneys, assistant county managers, and departments that are not responsive to community needs and appear to be extremely wasteful. And that's just the tip of the iceberg. Citizens have no idea of the waste, duplicity, and excessiveness that is part of this government. There is no transparency—and our county commissioners have no idea what transpires in county hall—they are just starting realize it, but it might be too late.

Lessons Learned

Lessons learned from this experience include:

- Build relationships.
- Don't try to be all things to all people.
- Provide evidence of the organizations impact on the community.
- Remember who you are serving.
- Treat all community members the same.
- Be honest and realistic—don't make promises you can't deliver.
- Listen.
- Consider the importance of collaborating with other county departments and the community.

Debbie Curtin passed away on August 11, 2008. Team Metro—the department that she created and nurtured—was killed off on September 30, 2008. Both are dearly missed by staff and residents of communities that benefited from government for the people.

Wait, There's More!

On July 15, 2009, the mayor of Miami-Dade County released his 2009–2010 budget proposal. Among the many items listed was the merging of the Office of Neighborhood Compliance with the Building Department, and the elimination of forty-five positions from the ONC. Of course, this is just a small percentage of the 1700-plus jobs that are on the table to be chopped, but in essence it cuts out the heart of what was left of Team Metro. The budget also effectively removes the outreach component from county departments. The GIC, the department that allegedly assumed Team Metro's outreach activities, is also eliminating its newly acquired outreach positions. So after fifteen years of attending homeowner association meetings and a host of other gatherings, the bridge between citizens and local government is gone. Talk about turning back the hands of time.

There is no doubt that in this current economic climate government must revise operations. The excessiveness that resulted from the housing market's rise created a bloated government. We must eliminate duplication and reduce spending. Unless the cuts and adjustments are made in the areas that truly warrant reduction (excessive raises and high salaries in the top administrative positions and offices, take-home cars, executive benefits, supplemental pay, unchecked overtime, etc.), the problems will continue. However, in order to truly make effective change, local government needs to step back and decide what type of community is desired—one that has a government that makes decisions in a vacuum, or one that collaborates with its residents and businesses to truly assess community challenges and needs. In turn, citizens must step up to the plate and be active participants in their local government on a continued basis, not just when there is a budget crisis. This is an obligation in a democracy. After all, what good is transparency if no one is looking?

10

Eliminating Institutional Racism within Local Government

The City of Seattle Race and Social Justice Initiative

Elliott Bronstein, Glenn Harris,
Ron Harris-White, and Julie Nelson

Imagine a City

Imagine a city in America where race does not predict the quality of education you receive. Where race does not predict how long you will live. Where race does not shape your career opportunities or predict how much you earn. Where race does not predict your likelihood of going to prison.

That city does not exist. But in the state of Washington, the City of Seattle is committed to *becoming* that city—to achieve racially equitable outcomes in key life indicators, to end institutionalized racism in city government, and to create a community that is enriched by its diverse cultures, with full participation by its residents.

Seattle is the largest city in the Pacific Northwest. From the top of the iconic Space Needle (built as part of the 1962 Seattle World's Fair) you can look west to Puget Sound and the Olympic Mountains, east to the Cascades, and south to Mount Rainier. Seattle has a national reputation for being politically progressive, culturally diverse, and economically prosperous. At this writing Seattle's half-million-plus residents are about 66 percent white. Asian communities comprise 12 percent of the total population, African Americans 7 percent, Latinos 6 percent, and mixed-race 4 percent. It is a city of distinctive, vibrant neighborhoods, and the epicenter of economic powerhouses such as Starbucks, Amazon.com, Boeing, and Microsoft.

But take a closer look. Seattle in 2010 is no different than any other city in the United States. The city's social inequities mirror national trends, and

157

many communities are losing ground. Race influences where we live, where we work, how well we do in school, how long we will live, and the likelihood of our involvement in the criminal justice system. People of color in Seattle account for a disproportionate number of people living in poverty. In 2006, the poverty rate of Native Americans and African Americans was twice the rate for whites. People of color also continue to experience discrimination in employment, housing, education, public places, and law enforcement.

The history of Seattle reflects the complexities of the nation's ongoing struggle to achieve racial and social equity. Early trading relationships between Northwest tribes and European settlers soon gave way to armed conflict, usurpation of land, and the establishment of tribal reservations. Chinese, Japanese, Filipino, and other Asian groups succeeded in establishing strong communities, yet continued to experience periodic waves of repression, disenfranchisement, or expulsion. The most infamous of these was the forced relocation and internment by the federal government of approximately 110,000 Japanese Americans from the region in 1942. African Americans migrated to Seattle to escape Jim Crow conditions in other parts of the country. Once they arrived, they were forced to navigate a de facto system of restricted employment and segregated housing. Prior to the civil rights movement, African Americans and other people of color in Seattle were systematically excluded from higher education and many professions and industries. The current racial makeup of Seattle neighborhoods is a legacy of restrictive, race-based covenants and redlining that were common in Seattle until the early 1950s. In 1964, the voters of Seattle voted down a local "Open Housing" initiative by a margin of two to one.

The movement to end racism in Seattle is far from new. Since the beginning of white settlement in the region, organizations and individuals used legal, legislative, and social pressures to fight racial inequity. In Seattle, local efforts to achieve race and social justice have been an important part of our region's history and are a source of civic pride.

But the question remains: in such a diverse, progressive and prosperous city, why do all the key life indicators (income, health, education, criminal justice, etc.) fracture along a racial fault line—and more important, how can we achieve different results?

Within Seattle City government, several departments had attempted to address racial disparities in the community and access for people of color to city services. During the 1980s and 1990s, citywide diversity and cultural competency training had created a relatively diverse workplace, but they had done little to address underlying systemic issues. By the late 1990s, a handful of city departments had begun to focus on institutional racism. In 2004, Seattle implemented the Race and Social Justice Initiative to address these issues throughout city government. Seattle Mayor Greg Nickels called for the initiative at the start of his first term as mayor, after his experiences on the campaign trail revealed a racial chasm in residents' perceptions of city government.

Overview of the Seattle Race and Social Justice Initiative

In 2004 it fell to the Seattle Office for Civil Rights (SOCR) to implement the mayor's powerful, broad mandate. SOCR was a typical urban civil rights agency whose bread-and-butter mission was to enforce fair housing, employment, and other antidiscrimination laws within Seattle's city limits. SOCR was known in communities of color as a trusted partner, albeit a part of the establishment.

Working in consultation with the mayor's office and key figures in several city departments, SOCR formulated the following set of principles, which would influence the direction of the Race and Social Justice Initiative (RSJI).

- Focus explicitly on race and institutional racism. Although the initiative acknowledged other systemic inequities based on class, gender, ability, or sexual orientation, RSJI would train its lens on racism because of its centrality in Seattle's experience, and the breadth and depth of disparities based on race.
- Define institutional racism as "organizational programs, policies or procedures that work to the benefit of white people and to the detriment of people of color, usually unintentionally or inadvertently." RSJI would not be another diversity or cultural competence program; it would view itself as a successor to that work.
- Focus on root causes and solutions. Previously, government typically had responded to inequities—when it responded at all—by developing programs and services to ameliorate the effects of racism. The initiative would focus on changing the underlying system that creates and maintains inequities.
- Concentrate initially within Seattle City government. The first priority would be to "get our own house in order"; in other words, to address institutional racism within city government as a necessary first step before engaging the community more broadly. Only when the city felt the initiative had gained some internal traction would it expand the focus to address race-based inequities in the external community.
- Achieve results. Racism is a learned behavior that can be unlearned through analysis, strategic organizing, and intentional changes in policies, practices, and procedures.

- View the initiative as a long-term project. There would be no rush for a quick fix. RSJI would be planned and presented as an ongoing commitment to a new way of doing business.
- Be accountable to communities of color. RSJI's success would be measured by its results: racial equity in the lives of the people who live and work in Seattle.
- Use a community-organizing model to move the work forward. RSJI would concentrate on strategically developing critical mass among city employees, "widening the circle" of participants who understood the goals and strategies of the initiative and could begin to put it into practice.[1]

Beginning in 2005, all city departments developed and implemented annual RSJI work plans. The key elements of these plans were included in the mayor's annual performance evaluations of department directors. Each department created its own change team—a group of employees from all levels within the department that guided and supported the department's work plan implementation and RSJI activities.

In addition to working on department-specific issues, RSJI also required departments to work on a set of citywide issues:

- *Workforce equity:* Improve diversity of the workforce on all levels and across functions by ensuring equity in hiring and promotion.
- *Economic equity:* Change purchasing and contracting practices to increase participation by people of color.
- *Immigrant and refugee services:* Improve access to services for immigrant and refugee communities.
- *Public engagement:* Improve access and influence of communities of color.
- *Capacity building:* Increase the knowledge and tools used by city staff to achieve race and social justice.

The Seattle Office for Civil Rights was responsible for overseeing the initiative, including monitoring departments' progress and developing and coordinating citywide employee training. A coordinating team of five SOCR staff members met weekly to plan and implement the initiative. Just two of the team members were dedicated full-time to RSJI; the others made room in their already crowded schedules for the new assignment.

In addition to departmental change teams, the initiative introduced another important component: a citywide core team of up to forty people, representing most city departments. Core team members received intensive training on institutional racism, group facilitation, problem solving, and strategic action planning. Core team members worked with change teams, department managers, and line staff to implement the initiative.

The RSJI subcabinet, which consisted of department directors and/or designates and the mayor's staff also played a key role in the initiative's organizing structure. The subcabinet developed proposals to address systemic issues and served as a forum for sharing RSJI best practices.

There was no roadmap for this work. No city in the United States had ever attempted a comprehensive antiracism initiative of this size and scope. The coordinating team drew on the wealth of organizing tools, resources, and knowledgeable people both in Seattle and across the country to develop its own model for action. For capacity building, RSJI organizers relied heavily on the work of three national organizations with deep antiracism teaching experience: The People's Institute, Crossroads, Inc., and Western States Center.

The initiative had one big advantage: a captive audience. A mandate from the mayor meant that departments could not simply refuse to implement the initiative. Employees who attended antiracism training could not walk out with impunity. This was work time after all, and participants were answerable to their supervisors, who were responsible to their directors, who were responsible to the mayor.

Many of the city's twenty-plus departments actively engaged with the initiative from the beginning, even as the RSJI coordinating team worked to define RSJI's precepts, institutional structure, language, and implementation schedule. One of the departments that embraced the initiative early on was Seattle Public Utilities (SPU), which manages the City of Seattle's water, sewage, drainage, and solid waste (including garbage and recycling) services.

From Theory to Action: How RSJI Played Out in Seattle Public Utilities

Seattle Public Utilities (SPU) is the city's second-largest department, with a total of about 1,400 employees. About half of its employees are based in the downtown core; the rest work in the field, which includes the city's two watersheds located in the nearby Cascade Mountains.

With strong support from its leadership, SPU put together a committed change team consisting of both line staff and high-level managers; in addition, several SPU staff members also became core team members and brought their expertise back to the department. SPU's early and deep commitment resulted in the department's serving as a laboratory for much of the initiative's early work on contracting equity, public engagement, and service delivery.

Seattle Public Utilities: Training Laboratory

SPU's earliest contribution, however, was in capacity building—increasing the knowledge and tools used by SPU staff to achieve race and social justice, primarily through training. Although other departments had begun training earlier, SPU was the first large department to launch large-scale capacity building. The department agreed to pilot RSJI's newly developed training modules for all its employees, including an eight-hour training session that the RSJI coordinating team had developed based on the Public Broadcasting System's three-hour series, *Race—The Power of an Illusion* (RPI). RPI was used as a basic training curriculum for all of the city's 10,000 employees. Organizers had piloted the curriculum with change team members from various departments, but they had never presented it to large numbers of employees who knew little about the initiative.

The PBS program provided an excellent history lesson on the origins and evolution of American racism, and used concrete examples and interviews to connect that history to institutional racism. The integrity of the footage and the scholarship of the commentators are hard to dispute (not that a few training participants didn't try). RSJI organizers found that RPI challenged people's passivity—it convinced most viewers to want to change the system. When organizers began showing the series to city employees, people who were predisposed to supporting the initiative found their commitment strengthened; people who had never thought much about racism before often were shocked and moved by what they saw.

Seattle Public Utilities management's commitment to train all SPU employees was a breakthrough for RSJI organizers. As the training proceeded, however, it became clear that RSJI needed to develop a follow-up training module for managers and supervisors.

"We needed something that would prepare leaders within the organization to actually implement the Initiative," said Darlene Flynn, who leads RSJI's capacity-building work. "It wasn't just about educating people. Training was part of our organizing strategy for implementation, and we began to use organizing strategies to plan the training."

The basic antiracism training that emerged probed much deeper than RPI, and the roll out to SPU managers (from top executives to field crew chiefs) had more than its share of rocky moments. Over the course of several months, RSJI organizers refined the training; they also added a skill-building follow-up that introduced hands-on exercises to apply RSJI concepts to program and policy planning and implementation.

"When we started, we were prepared to make mistakes, and we did," said Flynn. "We tried to stay open to better training models and techniques, and we learned. Our only loyalty is to things that work."

ELIMINATING INSTITUTIONAL RACISM WITHIN LOCAL GOVERNMENT   163

The SPU training experience taught the RSJI coordinating team a number of lessons, including:

- It can be done. Large-scale antiracism training within a workforce is both possible and workable.
- Leadership matters. When executive managers make personal commitments and dedicate the organization's resources to this work, middle managers and line staff inevitably take the initiative more seriously.
- It is important to match the training with the audience and with the organizing goals. All city employees need a basic understanding of institutional racism and the mission of the initiative, but *not* everyone needs intensive antiracism training.
- Training is not an end—it is a means to the end. The goal is to transform how the city conducts its business by changing policies, practices, and procedures so that the outcome is reduced racial inequity.
- Training large numbers of people is resource-intensive. A "train-the-trainer" approach needs to be part of any large-scale capacity-building strategy.

"SPU's commitment gave us the opportunity to see classic organizational change dynamics play out before our eyes," said Flynn. "You had resisters, undecideds, and advocates from the very beginning. Those patterns are typical in *any* organization introducing a systemic change initiative. Recognizing that fact helped us realize the importance of internal community organizing strategies to increase institutional support for change."

Seattle Public Utilities: Contracting Equity

Contracting equity was one of the RSJI's original areas of work. Local governments have long espoused a commitment to increasing the amount of business and contracting that they do with companies owned by people of color and women. The City of Seattle, like other governments, has struggled to achieve real results.

RSJI organizers viewed capital expenditures as part of the lifeblood of a city. If government restricts circulation of funds to significant communities, it is not just those communities that suffer—it impacts the financial and social health of the entire city. Government restriction of funds to significant communities affect the communities as well as the financial and social health of the entire city.

SPU had begun working to improve its contracting program prior to the initiative. There was a need and desire to improve outreach to and utilization of women and minority business enterprises (wmbe), which SPU refers to as historically underutilized businesses (HUB). In 2003, SPU appointed Marget Chappell to coordinate SPU's HUB program. SPU was one of several large departments within the city to dedicate resources to coordinate its contracting work.

"You need to have a point person to oversee and report on all spending, and to provide tools to the managers with responsibility for spending procurement dollars," said Chappell. As a black woman and a former business owner, Chappell had a deep understanding of both business and minority communities and held strong views about the issues and the solutions.

"We knew there were a lot of barriers for people doing business with the city because of the *history*—the broken promises, the unrealized expectations, the disconnect between what government said and what it did. The task was to overcome that legacy, rebuild trust, and reengage community businesses— and it is *still* a struggle," said Chappell.

She began by educating herself on every aspect of the contracting/purchasing process—both in SPU and within other city departments. Where and how did the city spend its money? What contracting processes did the City use? Which businesses were successful?

In 1998 Washington State voters approved Initiative 200 (I-200). Modeled after California's Proposition 209, I-200 banned the use of racial preferences in contracting and hiring by public sector entities. In the wake of I-200, the percentage of the City of Seattle's contracting dollars to wmbe firms had plummeted from approximately 30 percent to 6 percent—especially to businesses owned by people of color.

Chappell's in-depth research led to some key conclusions. The city's own contracting policies and procedures prevented the very equity to which Seattle aspired:

- Paperwork to register as an HUB was burdensome to small businesses.
- The cost of participating in the program was prohibitive. Businesses with narrow profit margins or lower cash flows had no way to gauge their likelihood of success, and, depending on the scope of the project, responding to requests for proposals could be very expensive.
- City purchasers were resistant to change. They tended to do business with the people they had always done business with.
- Institutional inertia allowed city contracts to take on the shape of their contractors. Over time, contracts tended to resemble the specific services provided by the current contractor. Without a truly competitive process, the city had no way to know if a price or a product was competitive.

ELIMINATING INSTITUTIONAL RACISM WITHIN LOCAL GOVERNMENT   165

Chappell's first action was to institute a new reporting system that reflected SPU's spending for contracting. The report showed a stark reality: almost 95 percent of SPU's contract spending went to white-owned businesses. HUBs shared the remaining 5 percent.

Then she developed and convened a series of meet-and-greet events for SPU purchasers to sit down and talk with local HUBs. Chappell made clear the expectation that both purchasers and businesses would follow up with one another after the event. "I made sure that the businesses brought formal profiles to the meetings that showed their scope of work, plus references. I wanted our people in SPU to see that these companies are competent, dynamic operations, and that it is in the city's interest to do business with them."

She focused her efforts on "lower-hanging fruit"—subcontractors such as office suppliers, carpenters, electricians, and landscapers. After the next bidding cycle, Chappell checked back with SPU's contractors and with companies that had shown interest in participating with the city. Had the company applied to participate in the city's vendor program? If so, did it receive a contract from a general contractor? And did the business actually receive dollars via a subcontract and make money on the relationship?

SPU's dedicated, multipronged approach to contracting equity eventually began to yield results. Some purchasing units increased spending with businesses owned by people of color. The utility also developed working partnerships with other large institutions, such as Seattle Public Schools, the Port of Seattle, and the Seattle Chamber of Commerce. Together the group has lobbied the state of Washington to change contracting requirements for public works to create more opportunities for like-sized businesses to compete with one another and for smaller businesses to compete well.

Most important, SPU's decision makers became more knowledgeable about HUBs and the importance of including them in the utility's overall purchasing strategies. Each branch of the utility formed a HUB action team that met regularly to monitor and analyze their purchasing and contracting patterns.

"It's a long, slow process," said Chappell, "But I am full of hope because I believe we are moving in the right direction."

Seattle Public Utilities: Outreach and Public Engagement

Outreach and public engagement was another major focus of RSJI. The City of Seattle was famous (or infamous) for its "Seattle Process," in which city employees would convene public meetings to "invite resident comment" multiple times, though not necessarily at the right time, early in the process and prior to plans' development. Since outreach and engagement took place so late in the process, how would comments influence the plan? The lack of

166   E. BRONSTEIN, G. HARRIS, R. HARRIS-WHITE, AND J. NELSON

early outreach and engagement was especially scorned within communities of color, who felt completely cut off from the city's decisions and practices. RSJI's goal was to improve access and influence of communities of color on city government—and, by extension, improve access for everyone.

Michael Davis's work on public engagement also predated the initiative—by about twenty years. Davis is a planning and development specialist focusing on service equity, but his first job as a city employee in the 1980s was to manage SPU's recycling, streetside litter, and food waste programs. He installed Eco-Village displays at summer fairs, with hands-on demonstrations about water quality and conservation.

"Before that we used to take the standard 'brochures-on-a-table' approach to outreach," Davis remembered. "The Eco-Village was different. We actually had displays of low-flow toilets and CFL bulbs, we gave away shower heads, vegetable seeds. . . . And it worked."

Yet he noticed something: no people of color. As an African American man, Davis wasn't happy. "I felt I needed to do something about that. And I think others began to feel that too."

By the mid-1990s, Davis had begun to partner with a variety of community-based organizations to create a different model for environmental outreach. SPU would train community members to display and talk about conservation, recycling, and water quality. SPU would pay them stipends to conduct information sessions, and would support them with materials, giveaways, consultation, and other funding.

Over time, the project proved successful—so successful that Davis and his coworkers in the Environmental Justice Network in Action began to use that model in all their outreach work. This occurred long before the emergence of RSJI, which provided the opportunity for the rest of SPU and other city departments to use a similar model.

"It was hard for us to partner with other divisions because they had no understanding of the equity framework we were using," said Davis. "Project managers who needed to do some outreach would call us at the last minute frantic for a list of names to call—or they wouldn't call at all, and then become angry when community people wouldn't go along with the city's plans. RSJI became a mandate for us to formalize the institutional values and common understanding of community partnership."

Many employees knew the public engagement system was broken, and they were frustrated. RSJI gave SPU employees the opportunity to learn that it "wasn't just them." It was an institutional problem, and there were structures and tools that could begin to change how government worked in this area.

Michael Davis believes—and the initiative echoes this belief—that city

ELIMINATING INSTITUTIONAL RACISM WITHIN LOCAL GOVERNMENT   167

government benefits when the whole community is better informed and more engaged. Under RSJI, the model that he and SPU began to experiment with in the mid-1990s now became official policy—not just within SPU, but across the entire city.

"The challenge is how to achieve that. We are trying to leave behind that model of one size fits all plus make symbolic gestures for communities of color," said Davis. "The job is to be much more intentional about identifying communities' different needs. Then we can ask ourselves, 'How does that help us achieve greater equity and impact?' It's not enough for frontline staff to get it—it takes a systemic approach with commitment, direction and support from top and middle management."

"A department may not have the capacity to create an Eco-Village, but perhaps it can expand its avenues to reach out to various groups, and also change the way people carry themselves when working with different communities of color," said Davis. "I'll be honest—we are still struggling to implement this. The advantage of the initiative is that we're finally having conversations throughout city government about what works and what opportunities exist. That wasn't there before. It's huge."

Seattle Public Utilities: Achieving Service Equity

A city's racial and ethnic composition and its service levels are closely linked, both in reality and in public perception. City of Seattle employees often talk about the "north end" and the "south end." It's unofficial shorthand for summarizing Seattle's racial and economic fault lines: from downtown north the neighborhoods are both whiter and more prosperous. South of downtown, the city is far more ethnically diverse and much less middle class. Perceptions follow the shorthand—for example, that the north end receives better services, while south end residents get a shrug of the shoulders.

When SPU began to implement the RSPI, its service managers realized that they did not know how true those assumptions actually were. For example, was the city making capital investments equitably across neighborhoods? That was hard to tell, because long-term spending often extended across many years. Managers soon realized that "Where does the money flow?" was the wrong question. They decided instead to scrutinize the bottom line of SPU's work: service delivery levels in different neighborhoods.

After all, SPU already routinely collected good statistics on its three core services: water, sewage, and garbage collection. Managers would simply run that data through a different filter—one based on the racial profiles of various Seattle neighborhoods.

SPU's statisticians and number crunchers went to work. They developed models that tied service levels to demographics, matching their data with the U.S. Census's census block group (the smallest geographic unit from which racial and income information can be extracted) to see if there was a correlation.

The service equity study team chose three specific measures to study: water outages, sewage backup, and missed garbage pickups. They found correlations everywhere they looked—not necessarily huge discrepancies, but statistically significant patterns.

Then they looked for possible explanations that were not based on race or income. They examined the underlying service infrastructures, such as differences in pipes and soils throughout the city that might affect water outages. Sometimes these explanations were plausible. But RSJI forced SPU managers to a critical recognition: it didn't matter if they could "explain" service disparities. What mattered was ending the disparities themselves.

The utility directed its service managers to follow up on the study's results. In the solid waste department, for example, SPU happened to be in the middle of renewing contracts for garbage pickup. SPU met with both contractors, shared information from the study, and instituted a monitoring process for missed garbage pickups in areas of the city where they'd found service disparities.

"We'd always tracked misses, but it used to be at the aggregate level," said Leif Anderson, a senior economist formerly with SPU who led the study's analysis. "Now we're following up on a quarterly basis at the more detailed level to ensure that service levels no longer perpetuate the old pattern. Contracts also contain new language allowing the utility to impose penalties for failure to meet the more detailed service levels."

Water managers knew it was fiscally impossible to replace miles of inferior pipes in whole sections of the city. So engineers got creative—they developed a practical proposal to add more shut-off valves to the water mains in those neighborhoods that experienced disproportionate water outages. Engineers hoped additional analysis would demonstrate that this and other system modifications can result in fewer households impacted by a system shutdown when crews need to replace a section of pipe.

"When I first took on this project, as an academic I naturally focused on causality: *why is this happening?*" said Anderson. "What the process helped teach me was the importance of the correlation itself. For all we know, many of those causality explanations are the result of past policy decisions—some of them long ago—that were themselves rooted in racism. Unearthing some of that information would make a great research project. But from SPU's perspective, it really doesn't matter why these disparities exist. What matters is to end them."

RSJI Citywide Accomplishments

In the end, moving RSJI forward began to resemble building a house. Much of the foundation work happened below the surface. Critical steps in the process yielded few visible results. Then suddenly the separate pieces were strung together, the walls stood up, and it started to look like a *building.*

When they began to conceptualize the initiative, coordinating team members faced a dilemma that is familiar to most community organizers. The initiative could hardly move forward until city employees received training; but political reality meant that implementation of RSJI could not wait until a critical mass of people somehow had "gotten it" through training.

Organizers decided to move forward on multiple fronts simultaneously by pushing capacity building (employee training), monitoring departments' annual RSJI work plans, and developing tools that city employees could use to apply RSJI principles to their day-to-day work.

In 2007, the city's finance department released its Budget and Policy Filter, a list of "best practices" criteria and a set of questions. The filter would guide departments through an RSJI analysis of a program or proposal. In the first year, the finance department required all departments to apply the filter to all new budget proposals to be submitted to the mayor's office. A year later, RSJI organizers introduced a revised version of the filter (now called the Racial Equity Toolkit) to planners and managers throughout city government. By 2010, departments had begun to use this tool to analyze the race and social justice implications of a wide variety of budget proposals, programs, and policies.

Since 2005, RSJI has resulted in other significant policy and program changes within Seattle city government.

- *Translation and interpretation policy:* A comprehensive translation and interpretation policy was created in 2007 as part of a strategy to improve immigrants' and refugees' access to services. All city departments provide essential translation and interpretation services for non-English-speaking customers.
- *Outreach and public engagement policy:* The city created an online Inclusive Outreach and Public Engagement Toolkit for departments' use. Departments created internal teams to implement the new approach and to document strategies that worked.
- *Contracting equity:* The city has improved its process and increased opportunities to compete. From 2003 to 2007, the city doubled the percentage of contracting for nonconstruction goods and services with women- and minority-owned businesses. The city exceeded its 2007 goal

by more than 40 percent. Despite these increases, results were not uniformly positive. Use of African American, Latino, and Native American business enterprises did not increase substantially, and became a focus of follow-up contracting efforts.

- *Workforce equity:* The city introduced new rules for departments to follow for temporary "out-of-class" assignments, which was an area of huge concern for many city employees. In 2010, the city was considering other upward mobility strategies for employees in low-wage occupations.
- *Capacity building:* By September 2009, close to 75 percent of all city employees had participated in RSJI training. In 2010, the Seattle Police Department and the Seattle City Attorney's Office, which had been slow to implement the initiative, organized change teams and introduced training based on *Race—Power of an Illusion* to their employees.
- *Other significant changes to business operations:* Under RSJI, departments have implemented significant changes to their administrative operations and programs. For example, the Department of Neighborhoods created a new RSJI category as part of its Neighborhood Matching Grant program to support actions in the community geared toward achieving racial equity. The Human Services Department revised its funding process for nonprofit community agencies to make it more accessible for smaller organizations, including agencies that serve communities with limited English skills. SPU created a new Environmental Justice and Service Equity division to ensure that all SPU customers receive equitable services, as well as have access to SPU decision-making processes. As part of the region's Ten-Year Plan to End Homelessness, the Office of Housing and the Human Services Department crafted a fundamental shift in the city's housing and shelter policies to acknowledge racial disproportionality in homelessness, and to focus efforts on people with the greatest housing needs.

The Next Phase: Extending RSJI to the Larger Community

In 2008, the initiative underwent a thorough assessment to measure progress and make recommendations for the future. The following year, the city announced "the next phase" of RSJI. In addition to continuing to address racial disparities within Seattle city government, the initiative also began to address fundamental race-based disparities in the larger community by developing partnerships with other key institutions, including the public and private sectors.

In 2009, RSJI's goals were reframed to include the original focus areas and to add an external component:

- End racial disparities internal to the city: Improve workforce equity, increase city employees' knowledge and tools, and increase contracting equity.
- Strengthen the way the city engages the community and provides services: Improve outreach and public engagement, improve existing services using RSJI best practices, and improve immigrants' and refugees' access to city services.
- Eliminate race-based disparities in the broader community.

The third point represents the ultimate goal of the initiative. To address race-based disparities in the community, the initiative created the RSJI Community Roundtable, a leadership forum on race and social justice composed of more than twenty organizations representing key public institutions and social justice leaders from the Seattle area. All members work to address institutionalized racism within their own organizations and are committed to collaborating across organizations. The Roundtable is charged with developing a shared vision and a collaborative action plan to achieve racial equity.

The RSJI Community Roundtable selected public education as its primary focus to end race-based disparities. As part of this effort, in 2010 the city asked departments to identify their own areas of impact on disparities in education and to develop strategies for change.

Politics and Opportunities

In the fall of 2009, RSJI weathered an unexpected and dramatic transition: a change in the City of Seattle's political leadership. That August, two-term mayor Greg Nickels lost his primary bid for a third term. The two remaining candidates for mayor were political newcomers who were unfamiliar with the initiative.

The initiative viewed this development as an opportunity to extend the mandate for RSJI within city government. RSJI coordinating team members arranged briefings on RSJI for both mayoral candidates. The candidates welcomed the information—both of them were fielding questions from members of the public about the initiative at forums across the city and realized that RSJI had significant support in the community.

Coordinators also met with key city council members to broach the idea of a council resolution of support for RSJI. Seattle City councilmember Bruce Harrell agreed to sponsor a resolution in November 2009. The resolution, which passed unanimously, accomplished more than simply affirming general support for the initiative: it also established a specific role for the council to monitor departments' progress on an annual basis. In addition, Councilmember Harrell joined the RSJI Community Roundtable as a formal representative of the city's legislative branch of government.

172 E. BRONSTEIN, G. HARRIS, R. HARRIS-WHITE, AND J. NELSON

After Mike McGinn was sworn in as Seattle's new mayor in January 2010, he quickly embraced the initiative. The mayor and his staff, many of whom had not previously served in Seattle city government, scheduled two days of training to familiarize themselves with RSJI. That spring, Deputy Mayor Darryl Smith instituted inclusive outreach and public engagement policies that were aligned with RSJI, and the city began using the Racial Equity Toolkit as part of its long-range neighborhood planning process in several city neighborhoods.

In June 2010, city council committees held public council meetings for departments to report their midyear progress on the initiative. As the mayor grappled with significant revenue shortfalls in 2010/2011 caused by the severe nationwide recession, he also made it clear to departments that he expected them to use the Racial Equity Toolkit to analyze the impact of budget reductions on both the public and city employees. Due to the severity of the budget shortfall, it was clear that there would be RSJI impacts, but by using the toolkit, city staff would be more likely to develop strategies to mitigate the impacts of those cuts.

Lessons Learned: A Model for Other Cities?

The City of Seattle Race and Social Justice Initiative is still a work in progress. Its accomplishments are real, but their reach remains limited. At this stage of the initiative, it is still difficult to step back and assess successes, failures, and ongoing challenges.

Nevertheless, a few lessons have emerged for RSJI's organizers who for the most part have worked together on the initiative since its introduction.

Necessity of a Shared Vision

RSJI's coordinating team spent many early meetings arguing the scope, components, and timing of the initiative. It wasn't always pretty. But the group emerged from that process with clearly defined mission, goals, and plans. From that point on, team members resisted the temptation to give in to so-called scope creep. Much of their resolve was buttressed by political realities: as a government project, RSJI had to remain realistic and achievable. But their resolve also was based on fundamental community organizing strategies of focus and discipline.

Relationships and Deliverables: Not in Conflict, but Working Together

Tension often emerges in antiracism work between the desire for deliverables or "products" and the primacy of relationships. Working within city government, RSJI organizers eventually saw this as another false choice, one that could pull city workers into endless debate. The way to change government is to generate a creative, complementary balance of both forces. In other

ELIMINATING INSTITUTIONAL RACISM WITHIN LOCAL GOVERNMENT   173

words, restore "relationships" to their key position within government, but never forget that you have jobs to do and services to provide.

Making Peace with the Power Structure

Antiracism work shares a number of organizational blockages often identified with other ideologically driven philosophies. Many people's vision of equity is linked with a parallel vision of consensus decision making, a sort of horizontal utopia where power itself is seen as racist and all participants have an absolutely equal say.

RSJI organizers took a different approach. Working within a large hierarchical institution, they recognized that "power" was neither good nor bad—it was simply inevitable. RSJI's goal was not to eliminate the hierarchical structure, but to use power to pursue and promote a race and social justice agenda.

Interestingly, RSJI organizers possessed little actual power themselves. They were a small committee within a small city department. Apart from the mayor's general mandate, RSJI held little clout of its own. RSJI could not order a department to introduce training to employees; it could not require a department to change a program or institute a new process. The reality of government forced RSJI organizers to use all the classic strategies of community organizing. They analyzed stakeholders and power dynamics; sought low-hanging fruit; built small alliances into larger partnerships; accepted setbacks as inevitable and necessary; and took advantage of sudden opportunities. They discovered how effective community organizing can be.

A fundamental question remains: "What difference will the Race and Social Justice Initiative make in the lives of city residents and businesses, as well as City of Seattle employees?"

Creating a shared vision and active commitment to racial justice is critical to achieving social change across our region. The Seattle Race and Social Justice Initiative represents a comprehensive effort to end inequities based on race and to reap the benefits of extending democratic governance. Success will be measured by what counts most: the racial equity in the lives of the people who live and work in Seattle. As we move forward on this long-term commitment, we recognize both the heroes who came before us and the leaders who will follow in our footsteps. The work we do is not just for now. It represents our contribution to those in the future—some of them children, some not yet born—who will admire our spirit, who will shake their heads at our mistakes, and who will build on our accomplishments.

Note

To learn more about RSJI and to download more detailed reports, visit www.seattle.gov/rsji.

11

A Case of Transformational Change

Making Sustainability
Real in the City of Olympia

Michael Mucha

Background

The City of Olympia is at the southern tip of Puget Sound directly between Seattle to the north and Portland to the south. Olympia residents enjoy a wonderful marine environment, mountains close by, parks, and access to nature. Olympia is also the state capital of Washington State and the hub of state government. Downtown Olympia has a progressive local flair, influenced by the presence of The Evergreen State College, which promotes democracy, inclusiveness, self-expression, and individuality.

After the United Nations Earth Summit on environment and development in Rio de Janeiro in June 1992, Olympia's city council and government entities were inspired to take action. The Earth Summit inspired governments to rethink economic development and find ways to halt pollution of the planet and the destruction of irreplaceable natural resources. Hundreds of thousands of people from all walks of life were drawn into the real process. The summit's message was that nothing less than a transformation of attitudes and behavior would bring about the necessary changes. Olympia's city council passed a resolution in February 1993 stating that current evidence indicates that global warming and ozone layer depletion as well as surface air pollution are occurring as a result of human activity. Although the rate of change and impact on Olympia are uncertain, the nature of likely impact on sea level, crops, water supply, energy, forest, and wildlife makes action prudent in spite of uncertainty. The council resolved that in the coming decade, the City of Olympia would respond to this prospect of global climate change by reducing emissions, increasing tree cover, and preparing for change.

In 2008, the city took stock and learned there are two things of greatest concern to Olympians. First, the projected two to three feet of sea level rise over the next hundred years will result in low-lying parts of downtown Olympia and its port being completely underwater during high tides. This threatens the economic, cultural, and social heart of the community. The second item is a threat to the city's natural spring-fed groundwater supply at McAllister Springs, at the mouth of the Nisqually Delta. Two to three feet of sea level rise would cause saltwater intrusion into a pure drinking water supply that currently serves a population of approximately 50,000 in Olympia and will be serving many more in the next hundred years. There is clear motivation to act and a realization that the city cannot act alone.

Climate change is playing out at the global scale, yet we can see how the fundamental dynamics trickle down to the local level. Increasing population and increasing consumption are occurring at the same time our resources are dwindling. The pressures of increasing population and consumption lead to reduced livability. The more governments do nothing about these problems, the more the public's trust in government's ability to provide value is eroded. These two competing trends close the margin for actions and make it more and more difficult to turn things around. However, leadership for innovative solutions that respect and care for people and planet by reducing waste, pollution, and consumption can create restorative actions.

One of the barriers to moving forward is fear. When confronted with something that overwhelms in life, humans often have two possible responses: (1) we retreat to the comfort of our beds, pull our blankets over our heads, and seek refuge in what is familiar; or (2) we go into denial. In the case of climate change, we see this manifested in people rejecting facts (denial and withdrawal): if the problem doesn't exist, we don't need to do anything. When sustainability is presented from a place of scarcity or fear (as can be seen in the popular press), denial and withdrawal run rampant. If sustainability is presented from a position of opportunity and leadership, responses may be different. Therefore, it's essential to lead sustainability efforts through what people value, particularly at the community level. Sustainability efforts go way beyond being "green." It is one thing to recycle, buy green power, and use hybrid vehicles. It is quite another to design and implement an organizational, cultural, and management strategy with sustainability as a central organizational and managerial principle. This is the beginning of the next wave of public management reform with the potential to restore and renew relationships among and between citizens and their governments—we might even begin trusting each other again.

Sustainability, then, is more than being green. It is transformational public administration. And, in order for transformation to happen in a government organization, sustainability has to be everyone's job and should not be rel-

176   MICHAEL MUCHA

egated to an Office of Sustainability, where sustainability is the responsibility of one particular person or organizational entity.

In any organization, transformational change takes place through initial major periods of growth, a plateau, a wake-up call, and then more growth. In 2004, Olympia's city council realized the city was at a plateau in their efforts to lead sustainability, and acknowledged that vision, plans, and intentions were not translating into tangible action. And mitigating the impacts caused by human activity would not be enough. Olympia needed to find a way to adapt to a new reality, and even more important, help shape that reality through micro decisions along the way.

The city manager formed a team of department directors, called the Sustainability Super Team, to ask why the city wasn't translating intention into action and how to move the organization forward with another transformational change. The Super Team learned there were three barriers to transformational organizational change with regard to sustainability:

1. Defining sustainability: Many people confuse the words *sustainability* and *environment*.
2. Inspiring the citizenry: People are not interested in sustainability if it makes their jobs more difficult; sustainability practices must make jobs easier.
3. Maintaining balance: Sustainability decision making had to balance often competing forces (people, prosperity, posterity, and planet), and employees needed tools to help make balanced decisions.

Step 1: Organizing Departments and Functions around Sustainability

The first step in responding to the three barriers to sustainability was to begin to organize city departments and functions around sustainability. The question was asked: "How do citizens experience the department?" Reorganization was designed around the responses. In the city's Department of Public Works (DPW), people experience the department through waste, water, mobility, and energy. Previously, the DPW had a fairly standard, "siloed" operational structure around functions: planning, engineering, and operations. Organizing around sustainability brought the functions into lines of business that deliver tangible value in terms of one aspect of sustainability. This created leadership and the focus needed to move toward holistic solutions for people. The DPW also refined their vision for a sustainable future involving all employees in a visioning process, through which sustainability was translated into "balance and harmony between people and nature." The department realized the im-

A CASE OF TRANSFORMATIONAL CHANGE   177

portance of the power of "and," and that they had to meet the needs of people and deliver high-quality services every day in an environmentally responsible manner. Employees at all levels of the organization easily grasped this concept and practiced it in their jobs whether filling a pothole or designing a thirty-million-dollar road project.

The DPW also recognized that if big changes were to be made in the community, they had to make big changes in how they viewed their role in city government. This role had to include cultivating relationships and facilitating change. They had to set the tone of a community in which people felt they belonged and were cared for, and that they had a voice in decisions that affected their lives. This cannot be done simply by changing the way one governs and administers; citizens will also have to change their behaviors over time, with the city employees as role models and facilitators to help move citizens to a place of empowerment and belief in their ability to affect change. This requires significant changes in employee skills, attitudes, and the systems used to get things done (the human resources manager, a member of the Super Team, responded to this demand for new skills for employees by developing new programs and training opportunities). The city also discussed organizational change that would eliminate certain departments.

Step 2: Develop Tools to Assist in Making Balanced Decisions

The second step in responding to the three barriers to sustainability was to develop tools to help employees make balanced decisions in ways that did not significantly complicate their jobs. The city worked with a student team from The Evergreen State College to design a decision-making tool that is interactive, helps find balanced solutions, is simple, visual, and user-friendly, and, most importantly, is on one page. The students, working closely with the Director of Public Works, created a Sustainable Action Map (SAM), which is now being used at all levels of city government (and by other cities throughout the nation and world).

The fundamentals of sustainability center on creating balanced solutions. Balance includes delivering a level of service citizens expect, doing it in an environmentally and socially responsible way, and ensuring the best economic choice for the long term.

SAM has three key dimensions that work together (Figure 11.1):

- NICE: The four key components of sustainability: the *N*atural, the *I*ndividual, the *C*ommunity, and the *E*conomy. All four of these components must be in balance to achieve a sustainable solution.
- SWOT: For any given action being considered, there are likely *S*trengths,

178   MICHAEL MUCHA

Figure 11.1 **Sustainable Action Map (SAM)**

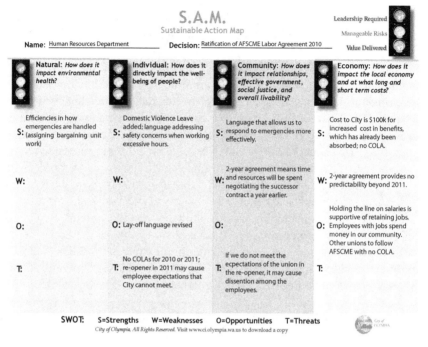

Weaknesses, Opportunities, and Threats. Each of these four components should be factored into a decision.

- The Stoplight: This system provides an indicator for how well a particular action achieves a component of sustainability. If it is green, the action provides value to that component (more strengths and opportunities). If it is yellow, there are risks, but they are manageable. If it is red, there may be some fatal flaws (many weaknesses and threats). This prompts leadership to consider innovative solutions to overcome these risks before the action moves forward.

SAM works through the following processes.

1. Identifying

Clearly identify the topic. Identify a clear topic, policy, or issue you would like to evaluate. Be specific, because this will help focus your discussion on the action most important to you. Write the action on the top of the form as a statement (e.g., "Building a three-lane roadway cross-section on Main Street," or "Removing glass from the recycling stream").

2. Brainstorming

Complete the framework on the form (get as many ideas as possible). Brainstorm the SWOT components: *S*trengths, *W*eaknesses, *O*pportunities, and *T*hreats. Start by asking the question, "So how does what we are proposing impact the economy?" Remember, impact can be good or bad. Strengths and weaknesses are things internal to your organization that you have direct control over. Opportunities and threats are things outside your control, and you must respond to them proactively.

Encourage the flow of ideas. Sometimes these will overlap. Start in one category that may lead to factors in other categories. Discuss those factors together and put them on the map at the same time so the team can begin to see the relationships and competing factors.

3. Distilling

Refine your brainstorming list to key issues. After brainstorming all the ideas, begin selecting what you believe to be the *most important* strengths and opportunities and the *most concerning* weaknesses and threats. For any issue, there should not be more than a few for each of the categories.

4. Evaluating

Determine how balanced your solution is. Step back and look over your prioritized list. What is it telling you? If a category has many strengths and opportunities, it is likely a *green light.* If it has some strengths, but also some weaknesses and threats you feel you can overcome, it is likely a *yellow light.* If there are some significant weaknesses or threats that you have not figured out how to overcome, it is likely a *red light.* One significant weakness by itself may warrant a *red light.*

5. Problem Solving

Find a balanced solution (all categories have a green or yellow rating). Focus the group's attention to the key issues that create *red lights.* Ask the question, "What can we do differently to turn this *red light* into a *yellow* or *green light?*" Some of those answers may take time to formulate. Create an assignment list for more research and agree to get together to discuss the solutions.

6. Move Forward

Clarify accountability for action that moves the topic forward. Once all your research is completed and you have a balanced solution, get commitments.

Decide who must do what by when to move the item forward. Pay attention to the specific actions necessary to overcome risks in the *yellow lights* and innovative actions that turns *red lights* into *yellow* or *green lights.*

SAM is a simple, yet powerful, one-page decision tool that guides the development of sustainable decisions. There are many potential uses for this tool. The three listed next are the most common:

1. *To optimize not compromise.* Asking the five SAM questions will help an individual or group think through an issue and formulate an outcome that is even more sustainable. When outcomes are sustainable, they contribute to the health of our communities.
2. *To select the most sustainable option.* While considering a variety of alternatives or pathways, the framework will help weigh the pros and cons and guide the most sustainable decision.
3. *To identify key issues.* Identify issues that are potential hurdles or enhancements as well as areas that could hinder or foster project success.

Our world is complex, and the choices we make always have trade-offs and opportunities. The power of SAM is that it does not just give one right answer. It helps make any decision more balanced. Use of the framework establishes a platform that encourages dialogue leading to trusting relationships and commitments to decisions.

The power of this tool is that it is scalable. You can use it at your desk or with a group. You can use the framework to do the following:

- *Find balanced solutions.* You can open up conversations around how to meet all healthy community needs when developing a policy, project, or action. When you meet all needs, you minimize conflict.
- *Tell a story.* You can frame how to communicate the information; ensuring users understand the relationship between seemingly unrelated things. By highlighting the cause and effects, citizens and others gain a better understanding of the project, moving the discussion away from a single issue.
- *Create openness.* You will give credibility to all points of view. It makes it safe to bring up all issues. Once the issues are on the table, you can discuss constructively.
- *Create focus.* You can boil issues down to key areas that need leadership attention to move from the current state to a future condition. This is what makes innovation happen.
- *Get things unstuck.* You can rely on the experience and judgment of the people in the room to address all needs and get things "unstuck" without analysis paralysis.

A CASE OF TRANSFORMATIONAL CHANGE   181

In the City of Olympia, SAM was used to guide major policy directions and make simple everyday decisions. SAM was fundamental in the development of a long-term strategy to help Olympia adapt to climate change and sea level rise, and address responses for the vulnerable downtown area. SAM was also used to develop a sustainable labor agreement with the American Federation of State, County and Municipal Employees (AFSCME), develop an employee wellness program, and the simple purchase of a new white board. SAM can be used for a wide range of organizational decisions, from the small, day-to-day things to major policy decisions.

Step 3: Provide Structure through Organizational Change

The third step in responding to the three barriers to sustainability is providing structure through organizational change. Putting systems in place that encourage sustainability helps reinforce its importance and helps to encourage a new way of operating. Ideals and a vision of sustainability are not enough. Systems and the organizational culture must change (Doppelt 2003).

In the area of systems, the City of Olympia focused on people resources:

- *New employment program.* The city launched a hire-for-attitude train-for-skill program, recognizing that bringing people into the organization who have an ethic toward sustainability and the aptitude to learn and adapt to a brave new world is most important. Skills can be trained on the job.
- *New employee orientation.* Every new employee of the city experiences an orientation about what sustainability is. They meet with the department director to discuss the vision of sustainability and the director encourages them to be innovators and masters of change.
- *Teaching sustainability.* The city offers four-day courses for those interested in studying sustainability concepts; from understanding what other communities are doing about sustainability to learning how to engage the public around sustainability. These courses provide advanced knowledge and understanding for the challenges ahead and opportunities to seize those challenges.
- *Cultivating leaders.* Confident leadership comes from within, and leaders must possess passion and desire. The city provides leadership development through education and training that awakens the soul.

Releasing Passion and Creativity

Having a good framework for sustainability and good training are foundations for leadership in sustainability. However, the hardest part is changing

182   MICHAEL MUCHA

roles, particularly of managers. Setting employees up for success is a crucial element to making the shift to more balanced solutions. Employees must feel they can meet their strong internal commitment to do a good job, but not as if they need to make sacrifices to be greener.

Finding balance is everyone's job. In fact, it is *the* job. It cannot be an extra activity or someone else's job. All employees at all levels must have freedom to advance innovative ideas.

Letting Go of the Reins

As public works director, I knew I had a department full of motivated, creative people. So what was preventing innovative solutions from coming forward? What I found out was that I was part of the problem.

Employees have an infinite number of great ideas that have the potential to create breakthroughs to new thinking. If every one of these ideas had to go to the director for approval, progress would be an agonizingly slow, focused more on bringing forward safe, noncontroversial ideas. Worse yet, if every employee waited for change to come from the director, the organization would be stuck in paralysis, churning along doing things the way they were always done before.

Therefore, I placed complete faith in employee judgment and creativity by getting out of the way so that they could lead. I did this by delegating almost all of the decision-making authority. I could then transition into a support role to remove barriers for employees.

However, this is not easy. It means moving forward and viewing success a little differently. Instead of viewing my role as being *relevant,* that is, being the person in charge with the good ideas, I had to view my role as being one of *significance,* that is, being comfortable in the background as a cheerleader for the vision and being a resource for helping to get things unstuck.

I needed to be accountable and to expect accountability from others, because the city manager was holding me responsible. My approach was to have a set of commitments that demonstrated what accountability looks like. I involved all employees in developing a document called "Our Commitments," and these points are reinforced ruthlessly, every day.

Purpose-Centered Leadership

To work for Olympia Public Works, everyone must be able to answer "yes" to the following questions:

- *Purpose centered.* Is what I am about to do a balanced solution? Is it consistent with our mission of being extraordinary? Will I do it in a way that honors our values of innovation, respect, and effectiveness? If the answer is "yes" to all five of these things, GO FOR IT!

- *Keep our promises.* Can I fulfill my "yes" commitment? If the answer is "no," ask for help.
- *Learn and grow.* If things do not go as planned (which will often happen if regularly going into uncharted territory), what new knowledge did I gain and how am I putting it to use?
- *Support.* Did we provide support to each other when things went bad? Spending our valuable energy looking for blame only keeps us stuck. Sometimes, managers must provide shelter from criticism.
- *Smell the roses.* Did we recognize the small successes along the way and enjoy them? If this is not done, work cannot be fun.

Under this form of accountability, employees are empowered to succeed for the department on their terms rather than being told what to do. This created synergy and meaning. Employees were now in charge.

Conclusion

The City of Olympia is doing extraordinary things on its path toward sustainability and is only at the beginning stages of the work. It is striving to implement sustainability principles (Doppelt 2003) that embody the Earth-Cat's (Hallsmith, Layke, and Everett 2005) five sustainability areas: social well-being, good governance, a vibrant local economy, efficient services and infrastructure, and a healthy, natural environment. The city is implementing transformative practices through four strategies:

1. Meeting human needs in the workplace and in the community
2. Leading by example
3. Balanced decision making
4. Engaging the community

One of the keys to the success of any sustainability program is to provide employees, citizens, and authorizing bodies (in Olympia's case, the city council) multiple portals through which to enter into sustainable practices, particularly early in the transformational effort. These multiple entry points include green practices, balanced decision making, performance measurement, performance bonuses, and social justice.

For example, the fire chief (a member of the Super Team) was highly skeptical of sustainability transformations and was initially motivated, by the city manager, to become interested because the department's performance mea-

184   MICHAEL MUCHA

sures as well as the chief's performance bonus were shaped by sustainability. The chief at first complied because it was a rational decision for him—his job performance depended upon it. Over time, though, he has become one of the strongest supporters and promoters of sustainability practices and transformations, as have the firefighters, because they have found ways, through sustainability, to do their jobs better, to make their jobs more satisfying, and to better serve citizens.

Is sustainability a portal through which public administrators can achieve the transformational effects we have sought for several decades? It sure seems that way. It is time for public administration as a discipline to pay more attention to the possibilities in these transformational practices and recognize the potential power of the movement that is bubbling up from local and regional levels and from other academic areas. Unbalanced solutions haven't "solved" our social problems—sustainability may not solve our problems and it may create new ones. Yet the potential is compelling. We may find practices and purposes that support economic viability, address social and economic injustices, lead to thriving and vibrant communities and individuals, *and* promote healthy ecosystems.

References

Doppelt, Bob. 2003. *Leading Change toward Sustainability: A Change-Management Guide for Business, Government and Civil Society.* Pensacola, FL: Greenleaf Publications.

Hallsmith, Gwendolyn, Christian Layke, and Melissa Everett. 2005. *Taking Action for Sustainability: The EarthCAT Guide to Community Development.* Montpelier, VT: Global Community Initiatives.

12

Think Global, Act Local?

A Short Story

Larry S. Luton

Jason Allen left the mayor's office with a song in his heart and a weight on his shoulders. Earlier that day he had walked eighteen blocks down the lower South Hill into downtown and up five flights of stairs in city hall feeling tired of facing the routines. He now knew that for the next eighteen months his work life would be anything but routine. He had been sitting in his cubicle—the 6-by-8-foot space bordered by movable, fabric-covered room dividers and fully filled with his computer desk, a filing cabinet, and two chairs that his boss, the director of planning, grandly referred to as his office—checking his e-mail, when Mayor Lightfoot's assistant, Allie, called.

"Good morning, Jason. The mayor wants to see you in her office at 10:00."

"The mayor? What's it about?"

"She'll tell you at the meeting."

As a somewhat nervous Jason sat in the waiting area outside the mayor's office, his boss, Mark Phillipson, came in. This caused Jason's anxiety level to go up a notch. Phillipson nodded a silent greeting, which did not reduce Jason's concern one bit, and sat across the coffee table from him. Phillipson picked up one of the city brochures on the table and began to thumb through it as if he had never seen it before. Shortly afterward they were joined by the mayor's assistant, Roger Aimes, and the director of public works, Gerry Adams. Aimes had run the mayor's campaign and was a very pragmatic strategist. Adams was a civil engineer who spent his first career in the U.S. Air Force, then started a second career with the city, beginning in the roads department and working his way up. Each in turn declined Allie's offer of coffee, and the conversation quickly focused on Sunday's Seattle Seahawks football game. Jason was not a football fan, but he tried to listen attentively as the others exchanged judgments about the quarterback's talents and the coach's strategy.

When the mayor's door opened, they all stood up. Out came the publisher

186   LARRY S. LUTON

of the local paper and the mayor, bidding each other farewell and thanking each other for taking the time to meet. In his charcoal suit and blue-and-red striped tie, the publisher looked every bit the conservative businessman with family ties to the local aristocracy that he was. The mayor was a picture of elegance in her gray pantsuit touched off with a red and silver scarf with a traditional Northwest Indian design.

In her office, the mayor greeted each of the directors, then Jason. At her invitation they all took a seat at the conference table next to the large window looking out over Columbia Falls's signature waterfalls, the urban park built around it, and the downtown skyline.

"Jason, you must be wondering what this meeting is about. I've been talking with Mark, Roger, Gerry, and some others for a few weeks about how the city can move forward on my commitment to promote environmental sustainability. I have decided to set up a task force that will prepare a sustainability action plan, a set of recommendations about how the city can operate with more attention to environmental stewardship, place reduced demands on resources, and become less dependent on fossil fuels for energy. Because of your personal concern about environmental issues and your background in urban planning and public administration, I want you at the center of that effort. I am asking you to accept a temporary assignment as the city's sustainability coordinator.

Without pausing for a response, she continued, "Mark has agreed to release you from your normal duties for eighteen months to support my initiative." Mark nodded his assent. "Roger and Gerry will work with you to secure a task force that includes people with expertise on the subject and represents a diversity of perspectives and interests." Roger and Gerry nodded their assent—Roger with his usual stoic demeanor; Gerry with a smile and a wink. "Once the members are selected, Gerry's assistant will work to bring the data management skills and technical expertise of his division to bear on the work of the task force. You will report directly to Roger on a regular basis, and he will keep me apprised of the task force's progress."

* * *

Returning to his office, Jason immediately called his wife, Courtney, to share the news, but he got her voice mail and remembered that she was in meetings all day; so he simply left a message that he had something important to discuss that evening. He could hardly wait to tell her, but he didn't want to miss her reaction.

After work, knowing that Courtney would be swimming laps at the YWCA before coming home, Jason walked to their apartment, put on his running

THINK GLOBAL, ACT LOCAL?   187

clothes, and headed out for his evening jog. On his way back, he stopped by the Real Foods grocery, picked up a pasta salad, some organic tomatoes, and a red wine that was on sale, then walked the last block home.

When Courtney came in the door, he had the table set, including a couple of candles, and the wine poured.

"What's with the wine and candles?"

"Didn't you get my message?"

"No. I didn't get back to the office after the meetings. So, what's up?"

"The mayor appointed me as the city's first sustainability coordinator today. I'm going to be released from my regular duties in the planning department for eighteen months to coordinate her sustainability task force."

"That's great, hon! . . . What will the task force do?"

"Write an action plan for how the city can operate in a more sustainable way—better environmental stewardship, reduced demand on natural resources, less dependency on fossil fuels."

"Wow! That's *great!* And just when you were wondering how long you could stand to spend your time fielding complaints from businesses and trying to keep traffic engineers from cutting down street trees. What will happen with the report when it's written?"

"I don't know. I'll find out more at a meeting with the mayor's assistant and the director of public works tomorrow."

"Who's on the task force?"

"We haven't chosen them, yet. They will have expertise on sustainability and come from different sectors of the community."

"What about Mark? Isn't he involved? How does he feel about your new assignment?"

"I don't think he's very happy. He was at the meeting with the mayor today and is going along with the idea, but I got the sense that he felt he could not say no."

"Oohh, what impact will that have on you when you have to return after the task force is done?"

"I'm hoping I never have to go back. After all, sustainability is not something that can be achieved in eighteen months. Anyway, let's celebrate! I've got an important and meaningful assignment. Besides, you know how crucial this kind of opportunity can be. We've been waiting for a chance to get my career in high gear and now we have one."

* * *

Roger began the meeting with Jason and Gerry's assistant, Tracey, by making one thing clear: "I don't want this sustainability thing to damage the mayor's

188   LARRY S. LUTON

chances for reelection. It's an important issue to her, but she can't do anything if she is not reelected.

"There are a number of ways we can protect her from blowback. First, the task force has to represent a broad base in the community—real estate interests as well as environmental interests, small businesses, transit, academic institutions, and state agencies (especially Ecology and Economic Development). There's a grant we can obtain from Economic Development to support our efforts. We'll ensure that energy interests are represented by having Richard Wellsworth from Northwest Power chair it. The mayor has already secured him for that role. He'll be joining our meeting shortly.

"Second, we need to open the process to anyone who wants to participate. We want to begin this project with a general meeting open to the public announcing the mayor's initiative and inviting participation. That meeting will also be a great way to flesh out a list of interested people. From that list we can begin to form work groups focusing on specific aspects of sustainability.

"Third, we need business and governmental institutions to have a specific channel of communication with the task force. We think that putting together a sounding board to meet periodically with the task force and keep them focused on practical solutions and economically prudent practices would address that need.

"Fourth, we need a proactive outreach effort to ensure communications with citizens and community interests beyond the open opportunity to participate in the work groups. We can't rely on people to volunteer to participate. We have to create forums and conversations wherever we can to engage with the community.

"Finally, we have to bring in speakers on sustainability that will gain media coverage and attract the public. The economic development grant will cover those costs."

Choking back his disappointment that so much had already been decided, Jason asked, "So what do you see as the role of the sustainability coordinator?"

"The mayor sees you as the central figure in making this work. It is your passion for sustainability that will give energy to this project. You will screen the applicants for the task force and present a list to her with your recommendations. She will, of course have the final say. You will write the ED grant—and the progress reports that the grant will require. You and Wellsworth will devise a schedule of meetings for the task force. You will also coordinate the meetings of the work groups, the sounding board, the outreach efforts, and the speakers from out of town. Working with the task force, you will need to devise guiding principles and decision rules and to organize the work to help move the project forward. You will be quite busy the next eighteen months."

Jason was not worried about being busy. He wanted to make sure he had enough of a leadership role to use this coordinator position to advance his career. He liked the design of the project and saw involving a wide spectrum of people as the right way to govern, not as a defensive strategy. He wanted the report on sustainability to change the way that the city operated, to change its organizational culture, and to lead the way toward a more sustainable community. Planning to work really hard, he thought he could make that happen; and if he made that happen, he could build a career based on that success.

Roger was explaining what resources Tracey and the public works department would bring to the effort when they heard Roger's assistant on the intercom announcing the arrival of Richard Wellsworth. Wellsworth was an impressive figure. Six feet tall, sporting an expensive medium-short haircut, he was impeccably dressed in a single-breasted dark blue suit, white shirt, and blue silk tie with gold diamond-shaped patches in diagonal lines. Entering the room, he greeted everyone by name as if they were all longtime friends. His handshake was firm, but not overwhelming.

Roger explained where they were in the conversation, and Richard thanked him for bringing him up to speed. Richard then expressed admiration for the mayor in taking this initiative and optimism about working with Jason to fulfill the task force's mission. The rest of the meeting was focused on setting criteria for task force membership and reviewing the process for inviting applications. Richard and Roger listed the names of some people they would encourage to apply. Jason also had some people he would like to see on the task force, but he decided not to name them at this meeting. Instead, he would contact them later to gauge their availability and interest. At the close of the meeting they all exchanged business cards and Jason and Richard scheduled a meeting the next week to discuss the economic development grant application. Richard told Jason to begin to draft the application and send him what he had prior to the meeting.

* * *

The first public meeting that Jason was asked to organize was described in the press release sent out by the mayor's office as an open meeting to discuss the organization of the sustainability task force. He was very pleased when about 200 people showed up at the meeting room in the downtown library to learn about the task force.

Energy levels in the room were high as the mayor opened the meeting with a statement about her commitment to sustainability and the importance of the work to be done by the task force. She saw this initiative as a central part of her agenda, and her charismatic leadership was a significant reason why so many people wanted to be part of it.

190 LARRY S. LUTON

People were excited to have such an initiative, and they eagerly put their names on lists to become part of the work groups, but they thought the task force members would be selected from the people who volunteered for the work groups. They did not know that the work of those groups would simply inform the deliberations of the task force. Instead of positioning themselves for a place on the task force by signing up for the work groups, they were volunteering to work *for* the task force.

When they found out that they were not to be part of the task force, some people were quite angry. Thinking that the task force would be a grassroots organization, they felt as if they had been deceived and placed into a subservient role. Those most upset by that confusion later decided not to participate because they felt their thoughts and expertise were not going to be appreciated.

* * *

Three months later the economic development grant had been approved and the task force members had been selected. Jason prepared a packet of information to give to the task force members at their first official meeting, which was to take place two weeks after an informal get-together at the Moosehead Grill, a popular downtown restaurant located in a remodeled industrial building and featuring regional microbrew beers on tap.

At the heavy oak tables they had pushed together to provide seating for eighteen, Wellsworth led the task force members through introductions and a discussion aimed at establishing guiding principles and hoped-for outcomes. The bar setting and the beer presented a façade of informality over a meeting that remained focused on the work to be done. The task force put together lists of guiding principles, process elements, and hoped-for results. Because a key purpose of the meeting was to begin building a sense of group identity, the lists were not composed of contentious items. The guiding principles included items such as "rewards proportionate to costs," "bridges economy and environment," and "builds awareness and support." The process elements list was also unlikely to engender opposition, including adjectives such as diversified and collaborative, and nouns like awareness, partnerships, and creativity. The first hoped-for result bullet point was "widely accepted." That list also included the terms "cost-justified," "coherent," and "actionable."

Jason was tasked with taking notes at the meeting and sending the members a draft statement of guiding principles the next day. His draft was emailed to the members for corrections, clarifications, and additions. Based on that feedback, he prepared a second draft for the first formal meeting, which was scheduled for the next month.

The first formal meeting took place in a conference room at city hall.

Unlike the Moosehead Grill, this was a sterile space with no windows. The walls were covered with the same fabric as Jason's office. At one end of the rectangular room, there was a whiteboard, which was covered up by a screen that dropped down from the ceiling. On it Jason had his computer screen projected to display the agenda.

The mayor opened the meeting by thanking everyone for agreeing to serve and remained for all the introductions, in which the task force members explained why they had agreed to serve and what interests, knowledge, and skills they brought to the work of the group. After the mayor left, the real work began. First, Jason presented the group with a matrix he had drafted to guide their work. He gave them paper copies and had the matrix projected on the screen at the front of the room. Having spent the previous weekend developing the matrix, Jason wondered whether he should have contacted Professor England, a member of the task force who taught policy analysis in Jason's MPA program, for some guidance or assistance. When that idea occurred to him, however, it was too late to benefit from it—besides, at that point he was already committed to the work he had done and could not risk being told to start all over, or even to make significant changes.

Jason's matrix anticipated having the task force members and the work groups evaluate each action item they might include in their final report based on the following criteria: whether it was an internal city operations policy or an external regulation affecting residents of the city; whether it was a short- or long-term action item; whether it dealt with reducing waste, greenhouse gas emissions, or oil dependence or with increasing energy efficiency or productivity; which aspect of the "triple bottom line" it impacted—economy, environment, or equity—and a number of feasibility issues (political, administrative, fiscal). It also contained a place for estimating the costs associated with each action item. His instructions for using the matrix described it as an exercise in systems thinking.

Following several task force members' expressions of appreciation for all the work and thought Jason had put into the matrix, Professor England said he shared the others' appreciation of Jason's work, but then he raised a question about how a linear matrix could be consistent with systems thinking, which he described as circular and recursive. "As I understand it, the fundamental characteristic of systems thinking is that it recognizes that everything is connected to everything else. Breaking these considerations down into each of these topics pretends that they can be addressed separately, that economy and environment, for example, can be treated as if they are discrete considerations, not overlapping and interconnected ones. We might want to use this matrix, but we need to recognize that it reduces our fields of view to the indicators listed and treats the whole as if it were simply the sum of its parts."

192   LARRY S. LUTON

Jason felt betrayed by this comment. After all, Professor England had taught him this analytical approach. Why did he teach it if he thought that it was a flawed way of analyzing policy options? But before he could fully process England's comment, Donnie Dawson, a former member of the state legislature, said, "My concern about this matrix is a practical one: Can we really expect to evaluate all of the actions we consider on over a dozen factors? How are we to estimate the costs? Even if we could theoretically do all this, can we do it in the year we have to produce an action plan?"

The task force generally agreed with Dawson's concern, but thought that the matrix could be a helpful tool for thinking through issues and proposed actions—at the same time acknowledging that they would be making many evaluative decisions without having the time to support those decisions with good data. They decided that the work groups would use it to put a common framework around their suggestions. Then the task force proceeded to modify the matrix by adding more elements. Jason did not know whether to be pleased that his matrix survived the challenges or concerned that its utility remained in question.

* * *

About a month after the task force began its schedule of four-hour meetings once every three weeks, it had its first meeting with the Sounding Board. Although the meeting was in the same conference room as usual, on this occasion, the screen was not lowered into position. The room was too crowded to give up the seat at that end of the conference table. So, everyone was expected to reference the large packet of information that Jason had put together for the board members to review prior to the meeting. Some had read parts of it and some had not. Their lack of preparation did not stop members of the board from complaining that they did not understand what the task force's mission was or what their role in its work would be. As the facilitator of the meeting Jason had to resist the temptation to suggest that if they had prepared for the meeting, they might understand better. Instead, he focused on providing, with some help from task force members, answers and explanations.

Once that phase of the meeting was over, the board members began expressing concerns about how the task force's action plan might affect their livelihoods. City department heads and local businesspeople found a common theme in admonishing the task force to make sure that it did cost-benefit analyses on all of its recommendations. Mayor Lightfoot and Richard Wellsworth were quick to assure them that no actions would be taken that did not make fiscal sense. Professor England, however, took the opportunity to hold forth on the difference between cost-benefit concerns and pecuniary interests, the first being a method of analyzing whether a course of action benefited a jurisdiction or community and the second a question of whether a particular business's profit margin might be affected. He also suggested that if the city were interested in promoting sustainability, the time frame utilized in any cost-benefit calculation would need to be measured in decades, not fiscal years.

To the professor's point about cost-benefit analysis being a way of assessing community or society impacts, not impacts on individual businesses, Susan Handy, owner of White Pine Coffee Roasting responded, "Well, I hope the community will pay for the costs."

The chief financial officer of the city, Garret Miller, expressed understanding of the time frame issue, but noted, "State law requires the city to balance its books each fiscal year."

Telling his wife about the meeting that evening Jason was concerned that economic interests appeared to have priority over environmental impacts. "I don't know, Courtney. The mayor and Wellsworth say that environmental sustainability is important, but they seemed quite willing to let fiscal and profit concerns place serious limits on what the task force will recommend. I think Professor England was right, but his comments didn't find much support and people seemed upset with him."

"Yeah, well I think the professor likes to stir the pot. His job doesn't depend upon the fiscal health of the city or a small business's profit margin."

"That's true, but I'm glad he raised those points. I hope that the task force's action plan will take economic concerns down a peg. We won't move forward enough on environmental concerns if economic interests retain control of the agenda."

"Well, I hope you don't side with him openly. He was your professor, but your career advancement won't depend upon his opinion of you."

"Don't worry. I'll be careful. Besides, no one seems interested in my opinions. They just want me to see that the task force gets its work done."

* * *

Jason's matrix, as modified by the task force, was introduced to each of the work groups at their first meetings. Meeting twice a month over the summer in the same conference room utilized by the task force, the work groups organized their thoughts and created lists of potential action items for the task force to consider. Only one of the work groups used the matrix as Jason had envisioned. The procurement group was led by an ambitious assistant manager in the city's solid waste division. He spent many hours outside of the work group meetings utilizing the matrix to present more than a hundred specific action items, most of which were his own ideas, not derived from the work group discussions.

194 LARRY S. LUTON

The other work groups each found their own ways of working around the matrix rather than with it. They developed lists of action items that were reflective of the content of their meetings, but they did not utilize the matrix to evaluate them. Work group leaders said it was just too complex to use. One common complaint heard from those who tried to work with the matrix was the absence of definitions and standard scoring formats for the criteria. That meant that similar scores on items might mean quite different things. Although city staff at the meetings might have been able to clarify meanings for the work groups, their input was often not welcome. One work group asked the city staff to refrain from attending their meetings; they felt that the city employees were trying to narrow the scope of what might be considered.

The water group got tangled in trying to determine whether they should provide support for the mayor in a controversy she had started by proposing new policies restricting water use. Her proposals—for rates that would have charged big users more per gallon and for restrictions on the times of day during which lawn watering would be allowed—had created a huge outcry from the city's residents. Even though that policy proposal was not part of the task force's work, the water group spent a lot of time and energy discussing it.

All of the work groups watched their attendance dwindle over the summer months. Meetings that were scheduled from 5 to 7 P.M. on workday evenings, when the sun was setting late and it was possible to enjoy outdoor activities well into the evening, required a serious commitment on the part of the participants. One work group chair decided to spend her own money on ice cream and other treats to encourage people to attend. The city had no funding for that kind of thing, but she decided that she just had to do it, even if it came out of her own pocket.

Some work groups were captured by special interests. The mobility work group's process for evaluating action items began with open discussions and wide-ranging conversations that took up most of the scheduled meetings. One meeting was consumed by a discussion of whether it would be legal for the city to place a preference for local vendors in their purchasing standards. Another included an extended argument in favor of making biofuels in your own basement. Several involved lengthy promotional pitches by members of a local electric car club.

At their last meeting, large sheets of paper had been attached to the walls in the room. On those sheets were listed action items that the group had discussed in their earlier meetings. Each person in attendance was given five colored dots to place next to their favorite action items. The dots represented their votes, and they were allowed to use all of the dots on one item or to place dots on up to five different items. Since participation was wide open, a contingent of electric car enthusiasts was able to utilize their dots to ensure that several items promoting the use of electric cars were forwarded to the task force for its consideration.

The work groups submitted their results to Jason prior to their chairs' formal presentation of them to the task force at its September meeting. So he knew before the task force did what a disparate set of analyses and presentations they would see. The procurement work group co-chairs limited their Power-Point presentation to a top-ten list, plus twelve "low hanging fruit" items. And although the built and unbuilt environment group co-chairs focused on a top-twenty list, they presented 322 action items. The water group presented twenty-five more. In their PowerPoint presentation the transportation and mobility group scrolled seventy items at an unreadable speed to indicate the editing they had done to reduce their presentation to a top twenty-five list.

Jason held a debriefing meeting with the work group chairs the week after they presented their work to the task force. At that meeting, he reiterated the appreciation of the task force for all the time and effort they had given over the summer and presented them with an official invitation from the mayor to a reception in their honor that would follow the presentation of the task force report to the city council.

All of the work group chairs at the debriefing meeting agreed that the lack of definitive direction was frustrating and the amount of work unexpected. Some complained that too few people from the business community participated. Callie Cummins, one of the co-chairs of the built and unbuilt environment work group was very unhappy. "Why did you begin with a general public meeting that seemed to invite all who showed up to be part of the task force, then choose an elite set of members for the task force and relegate us to work groups? It's not fair that the task force gets all the credit and we did all the work. Oh yeah, and I won't be at your reception."

Jason did not understand the complaint about how the task force was selected. He thought it was quite clear from the beginning that it would be a select group appointed by the mayor. Moreover, that was done and could not be changed. So he skipped over that complaint and tried to address the complaint about getting credit. "I hope you'll change your mind about the reception. The mayor and the task force recognize and appreciate all the work you did, and they want to honor you with a reception. You'll also be given credit in the report. Every idea that your work group submitted, and the prioritization that you did, will be included."

With her arms crossed and her eyes burning holes in him, Callie said, "Yeah, thanks."

* * *

196 LARRY S. LUTON

It took several meetings for the task force to begin to sort out how they were going to get from the 800 or so action items that had been offered for their consideration through the various forums, work groups, outreach efforts, and so forth to its final report. They also added over forty new ideas that had not come from public input. In an effort to make the report more readable, they worked for a couple of meetings at identifying themes with which to organize the report. At one meeting they identified the themes as stewardship, land use, waste management, connectivity, localization, renewable energy, and efficiency, but they were not satisfied with this long list and resolved to find broader themes. The primary accomplishment at the next meeting was to identify restructuring, resource stewardship, and resiliency as the "three Rs" they might use as organizing themes.

While they were struggling with how to organize their recommendations, Jason was working on a new matrix to capture all of the action item suggestions and categorize them according to their sources, whether they were among the top-ten items as presented by a work group, and which of the three Rs they related to. For the November meeting of the Green Team (representatives of city departments) he added columns that allowed the action items to be labeled as follows: already done, can't do, could do, could do better, could do if, or pass for now.

It was these added columns on which the Green Team focused. They could not have cared less about which of the three Rs the action items related to or what the sources of the items were. Knowing that the work groups' top-ten lists would get more of the task force's attention, they made sure to evaluate those items as to their feasibility.

In the list of hundreds of action item suggestions, they found sixty-four that the city was already doing, and a dozen that they categorized as "can't do"—most because they were not within the city's authority and some because they had been tried before and failed. Others they simply did not like.

George Pearl, from the human resources office, began the discussion of the task force proposal to incorporate environmental stewardship criteria into evaluation procedures for all city employees. "This action item will open a huge can of worms. To do it will require changes in both the union contracts and civil service rules."

Others piled on. "I don't like the idea of adding criteria to my annual evaluations." "Aren't we being held accountable for enough things? Why should sustainability be placed in our laps, too?" "Shouldn't responsibility for incorporating environmental stewardship into city operations be placed on management?"

Jason explained, "The task force added this item themselves. They said that incorporating stewardship into city operations required not only encouraging city employees to ride the bus or carpool; it also required every employee to think about environmental stewardship and find ways to bring that value into their daily work. They said that in order to get that kind of change it had to be measured and the measures had to part of the employee evaluation procedures. You will note that it covers all city employees, including management."

The Green Team decided to mark that action item as "pass for now."

* * *

When the mayor's task force met to revise and adopt their action plan, Professor England noticed that the proposal to incorporate environmental stewardship into employee evaluations was no longer in the list of action items to consider for inclusion in the plan. "What happened to it?"

Jason explained, "The Green Team didn't like the idea very much."

"Well that's too bad. I think it needs to remain in our plan."

Wellsworth added his support. "If we don't measure it, things won't change. If the measures don't have any way of affecting employee behavior, it won't get done."

The task force quickly reached a consensus that the stewardship in evaluations recommendation would remain in the plan.

Consensus was not reached as easily on a number of other action items. Sherrie Miller, CEO of Columbia Regional Transit Agency, the agency that ran the bus system, raised an objection to the action item recommending fixed-route transit corridors as a way of encouraging denser residential and business development along the corridors. "It just doesn't work that way. We don't need to place such an emphasis on fixed routes."

Professor England responded: "Sherrie, do you have any evidence to support that claim? Everything I've read indicates that fixed-route mass transit works exactly that way. Once the real estate developers know where the routes are going to be, they invest in properties along that route. Condos and apartment complexes are built along the route to provide their residents with easy access to the transit system. Businesses also move in along the route because they know that customers will find it easier to access them. It's a specific version of location, location, location."

Used to getting her own way in discussions in her agency, Miller sputtered, "Bus routes do the same thing."

"No, they don't," said John Pattison, executive director of Inland Northwest Natural Resources Advocates, who was normally a voice for compromise. "Bus routes can be changed too easily for developers to be willing to invest along them."

Donnie Dawson, a former state legislator and current member of the Growth

198   LARRY S. LUTON

Management Hearings Board, weighed in, "But fixed-route mass transit is so capital intensive. Do we want to put so much emphasis on a system that is so expensive, inflexible, and will serve a limited part of the community?"

After working over the language of the action item, the task force was able to agree on the following:

> Support CRTA in its efforts to expand a multi-modal public transportation system that is clean, efficient, and user-friendly—particularly in 1) securing right-of-way for fixed-route rapid transit; and 2) aligning routes with corridors established in the city's comprehensive plan.

Sandra Odell, government affairs director of Columbia Home Builders and Realtors Association, objected that the proposed action item to "create denser population communities by amending land use policies and regulations to eliminate barriers and incentivize mixed-use, sustainable development" would punish private developers for building traditional single-family homes.

Pattison replied, "The idea is to provide incentives, not exact penalties. It would be kind of like the tax abatements the city has offered for developers who redevelop older buildings in the downtown area into condos. Maybe we should take out the word *create* and replace it with *encourage*. After all, the city won't create the communities; the developers will. We just want to promote denser population areas within the city. They are more energy efficient and support the use of mass transit. One of the biggest problems we have in increasing the use of mass transit is that we don't have neighborhoods with dense enough populations."

The task force agreed to replace *create* with *encourage*.

Then Wellsworth suggested that they also might consider avoiding the word *denser.* "People react negatively to the idea of denser population."

"How about replacing 'denser population communities' with 'compact communities'?" asked John Hill, an environmental planner from the Department of Ecology. The task force liked that idea, too.

Maria Perez, director of Citizens for Justice, raised a concern about an action item intended to raise water service fees. "If we 'incentivize water conservation,' won't that mean that people have to pay more for their water service? Especially if the rates are supposed to 'reflect the market value of energy.' Wouldn't that market value fluctuate rather unpredictably? What about the impact on the low-income population? Aren't we forgetting about the 'equity' part of the triple bottom line?"

Wellsworth responded, "One of the things we've discovered in going through the data is that water service has a huge energy component. To get water to consumers requires pumping it, and that takes a lot of energy. Our community has an average per person daily water use rate that is one of the highest in the country. We need to set conditions that reduce our consumption of water. That, in turn, will reduce our consumption of energy and reduce our carbon footprint."

Joining Perez in expressing concern about this action item, Odell offered another perspective. "Our low water rates are one of the more attractive aspects of living and working here. Many places lack the kind of water resources we have. Do we want to reduce our attractiveness to residents and businesses?"

England chimed in, "According to the climatologist at our forum this summer, as global warming increases, we are likely to become more attractive as a place to relocate. We have a good water supply and inexpensive energy rates. The milder winters that result from global warming will be seen as a plus by many. Our summers are wonderful now. Slight warming in the summer will not be much of a detractor. Still, the aquifer is a limited resource and the loss of snowpack in the mountains will reduce our water supply over time."

The task force decided to modify the water rate action item to read, "Equitably incentivize water conservation."

Dawson, the former legislator, raised a concern about the action item to "prioritize workforce development initiatives and partnerships that grow green jobs and green businesses." "What do we mean by 'green jobs and green businesses'? Is anything that reduces energy or water consumption or generates less pollution 'green'? Is a bicycle shop green? Is a used book store green, but one that sells new books and e-readers not? If Lowe's has human powered push mowers in their line of lawnmowers, does that make them a green business?"

Fred Knutson, the Department of Ecology representative, admitted that these were good questions, but that he hoped the task force would retain the green jobs action item. "There may not be a lot the city can do to grow green businesses, and what qualifies as green or not is not a simple question, but we ought to use our voice to move things in that general direction. Many of our recommendations are somewhat vague. They all have to be turned into action by others in the city. I think this is a recommendation we want to keep in our plan."

After some discussion, the task force decided to retain the language about green jobs and businesses, but added the phrase "particularly in the realm of energy efficiency" to keep it focused more clearly on aspects of sustainability that the task force was charged to address.

* * *

200   LARRY S. LUTON

Shortly after the task force agreed on a first draft of their action plan, Jason met with Mayor Lightfoot and her assistant, Roger Aimes, to provide an update and talk about getting a final version ready for presentation to the city council. She knew that some of the city council members had attended task force or sounding board meetings, but she urged Jason to have task force members meet individually with council members to gauge their positions on the action plan.

Aimes said it was already clear that two of the seven council members would oppose the plan. Nancy Edwards, an evangelical who represented the most conservative district in the city, had long expressed concern that the task force was not representative of the city voters. Bob Pearson, who also came from that district, had told many people that he thought global warming, if it existed, was caused by sunspot activity, not by humans.

Two of the council members could be counted on to support the plan. Steve Walker, a staunch liberal, and Richard Harrison, who was known for his support of environmental causes.

That left three members who could determine the outcome of the vote. The council president, Joe Sweeney, thought of himself as a progressive person, one who was open to innovation and change, but he had not paid much attention to the task force's work. He had never attended any of the meetings or public forums. A real estate developer who saw himself as a mover and shaker, Al Lockwood was an aggressive defender of small businesses but he also saw city government as having a proper role in coordinating the development of the city. The seventh council member, Mike Brown, had been appointed to the remainder of Mayor Lightfoot's term when she resigned her position on the council after being elected mayor. His political and policy leanings were not well known because he had never run for office. When he was interviewed for the appointment to the council, he had clearly indicated that he was not interested in running at the end of the term. That was one of the reasons he was selected, but it was becoming clear that he had changed his mind. He was really enjoying being on the council but had not yet tried to determine how much support he would have if he decided to run. Not an active member of either major political party, he had chosen to present himself as nonpartisan.

Mayor Lightfoot had to get to another meeting, but before leaving the room, she told Aimes and Jason, "Make sure you do the groundwork to get a 'win' on this one. Sustainability is a key to the future of this city and an issue on which I campaigned. We need to get the city council on board."

After she left, Aimes told Jason, "The mayor has placed a lot on the line on this sustainability thing. For better or worse, she is identified with it. We can't let it hurt her chances for re-election.

"We are going to make it as easy as we can for the council members to vote 'yes.' We will present the action plan to them and ask them for a vote to 'accept' it. They will not have to endorse it, just accept it."

"Keep me apprised of what you and the task force members learn about the positions of the council members on the action plan. I don't want any surprises."

* * *

The Tuesday evening prior to the city council meeting at which the task force report would be on the agenda, members of the local Tea Party held a meeting at Denny's restaurant. With an American flag in the background, Rebecca Polson called the meeting to order and led the group in the Pledge of Allegiance.

Next came a round of introductions, each person saying their name and a little bit about themselves or why they were there. "I'm a taxpayer." "I'm a concerned patriot." "America has lost its way." "Obama is a socialist and hates white people." "The GOP has lost its way." "Global warming is based on junk science."

After the introductions, Polson gave a short talk. "We're all here because we don't want to lose our country to the communists and the fascists who would take away our liberty. We need to take our government back. We have a president who wasn't born in the United States and a government that wants to take over all aspects of our lives, from our bank deposits to our health care to our right to drive our cars. In Columbia Falls, it is difficult to fight DC or the UN, but we can stop our city from becoming part of an international conspiracy. This mayor's task force on sustainability is something we have to stop. It has ties to the UN and a group called ICLEI that intend to clamp down on our freedoms by promoting the false idea that humans cause global warming. They are opposed to cows because they create methane. Where are we supposed to get our milk? They want to treat carbon dioxide as a pollutant. They want to stop us from breathing out. Well, we're going to stop them!"

* * *

The city council session at which Wellsworth was scheduled to present the sustainability action plan began, as usual, with each member reporting on some of their recent activities. Sweeney talked about his meeting with the police advisory committee, addressing his concern that the committee did not have sufficient authority and resources to examine police operations and reports of improper police behavior in an independent fashion. Edwards reported on her

202 LARRY S. LUTON

work with a Block Watch group, emphasizing the importance of neighborhoods' taking responsibility for their own safety. Pearson, reflecting on a meeting with a local nonprofit group, made an impassioned plea for neighborhood activism aimed at helping the less fortunate among us. Walker reminded everyone that the local public radio station was in its pledge week. Harrison made a pitch for people to participate in the upcoming "bike to work" week. Brown told a story about his visit to an elementary school to talk about citizenship. Finally, Lockwood reported on his participation with a Chamber of Commerce delegation to Olympia to visit with legislators and make them aware of issues and needs that were important to the Columbia Falls economy.

When it was Wellsworth's turn, he came forward in a nicely tailored suit that was the solid gray of an overcast day. Wearing a white shirt, the only splash of color was his blue–and–gray horizontal stripe tie. His PowerPoint presentation was projected on the large screen to stage left of the council members.

Wellsworth began by reviewing the process that the mayor's Task Force on Sustainability had taken, emphasizing that it was open, transparent, and involved over 500 people who provided about 800 discrete suggestions for action recommendations. He explained how the task force had sifted through the suggestions, focusing on things that the city could do, or could do better. "We were striving for stewardship and efficiency in all things." He concluded by describing the action recommendations of the task force as ideas that were worthy of further analysis, including cost-benefit analysis by city staff. "It will be up to the city to decide which of these recommendations to implement, and how to go about their implementation."

Council President Sweeney was the first to speak after the presentation was concluded. "We really appreciate all the work that you and the task force put into this report. Let's review the names of the task force members and have those who are here stand to be recognized. Again we appreciate your work. At the end of the day this is about the social and economic health of the community."

Pearson followed. "The founding principles sound very good, but it seems to me we're really jumping the gun here. Why are we taking action *before* the state and federal government move?"

Sweeney responded, "Hundreds of cities are taking action now. Thirty-eight states already have plans and another nineteen have legislation. We are not ahead of the game, we are just in it. This report ensures that we encourage sustainability and efficiency—that we do not create or retain barriers. It is an invitation to prepare well—to model best practices and to incentivize good decisions."

Edwards joined the discussion. "This all flows directly from the Kyoto Protocol. The UN thinks each person should have only twenty-six gallons of water a day. Once we open the door, we will have restrictive policies and regulations."

Harrison adjusted his wire-rimmed reading glasses so he could look over them, and explained in some detail how the sustainability report simply encouraged a direction in which the city was already headed. "Even if we did not package this around greenhouse gases, these are all actions we should take. This is a list of ideas that just make sense on their face. It's not about the environment *versus* the economy. Besides, all this report contains is recommendations. It is up to us to decide what actions to take."

Then the floor was opened to public testimony.

Mark Adams, a former state senator, was the first to the podium. "At first glance this appears to be a reasonable report, but I have a few concerns. First, the task force should go back and broaden its base with the business community. Talk with the people in the neighborhoods. We need to go slow on this. Haste makes waste. We need to be careful, especially in light of our current budget shortfall."

The Tea Party leader, Rebecca Polson, was next. "The premises of this report are based on faulty or at best incomplete science. At a recent meeting of climate change skeptics in New York City, there were thousands of scientists. Climate change is a myth. This report is one-sided and driven by a political agenda that comes from abroad. The Department of Ecology takes its definition of sustainability from the Brundtland Report.

"I believe in local control. You are implementing a UN agenda. Why should we take actions that will drive up taxes?"

Council President Sweeney interrupted. "There is no mention in this report of higher taxes."

"It will lead to that."

Sweeney asked, "Where did this stuff about the UN mandate come from? No one from the UN tells me what to do. Ecology does not tell us what to do. The EPA does not tell us what to do. This is a local document. It will be refined by the city council and what we decide to do with it will be assisted by the testimony at these hearings."

Councilwoman Edwards interjected, "This is all part of Local Action 21, which is part of Agenda 21, a global agenda."

Then Sweeney asked Polson, "Do you have a problem with energy security?"

She offered a curt response: "We have plenty of oil."

The next member of the public came to the podium and said, "I am against this sustainability thing. You are losing your authority. We don't want any more of that international stuff—or national stuff. How can we live on twenty-six gallons per day? Most of the toilets in our city are seven-gallon flushers. The report is packaged well, but the mayor's task force is sweet-talking you."

204 LARRY S. LUTON

"What about this 'conserve water everywhere' recommendation? To conserve something that you have a lot of doesn't make any sense. My son was in Europe, and they don't wash or change their clothes for a week. They stink. Do you want the citizens of our community to stink?"

The next public testimony came from a Unitarian minister who described himself as a supporter of the task force report. He agreed that "We do have a lot of water here. In global warming that will mean that a lot of people want to move here. Right now we use more per person per day than any community in the United States. We are on this earth together. Think about your grandchildren."

Seeing no one else who wanted to speak that night, Sweeney closed the council meeting by saying, "All we are being asked to do with this report is to accept it. There may be some semantic differences in what people think 'accept' means, but that is what we have before us.

"We will come back to this at the next meeting. In the meantime, we will take feedback by phone and email. We will also allow additional testimony at the next meeting."

* * *

The following Wednesday, waiting in the lobby of the newspaper offices to be called in to a meeting they had requested with the editorial board, several members of the mayor's task force discussed the Monday night city council meeting.

Knutson, the department of ecology representative, said, "Where did those people come from? I couldn't believe it. All that stuff about the UN. You'd think that we were delivered here in a bunch of black helicopters."

Dawson admitted, "They *were* pretty bizarre, but we are going to have to deal with them. They at least have Edwards and Pearson on their side. They might also affect Lockwood, and I hear that Brown is putting together a resolution of acceptance that spells out that by accepting the report they are not saying that they agree with it or will act upon it."

Odell said, "I think that would be ok. All they need to do is vote to accept it, no matter what that means."

England postured: "I don't know how we can be surprised that those ideas are being expressed. All over the country there are people who do not believe in global warming. Given the conservative nature of our community, we should have known that we would hear from them. I guess I was just surprised at the number of people who showed up to present that point of view."

At that point, the receptionist came to usher the task force members into a conference room to meet with two members of the editorial board.

THINK GLOBAL, ACT LOCAL?   205

Dan Porter, editor-in-chief, began the meeting by reviewing his understanding of the origins and purpose of the mayor's task force. Then he raised a question: "Why, if this is a mayor's task force, do you need to have the city council take a vote on it? Why not simply present it to the mayor?"

Dawson replied: "The mayor wanted this to be an inclusive endeavor. Making the kinds of changes the report suggests will involve all of city government. The city council needs to be part of the discussion."

Porter replied, "But couldn't it just be presented as an information item? Why ask the city council to accept it?"

Kirk Smith, a member of the editorial board who also writes a regular opinion column on the editorial page called "Sharp Points," wanted to know, "What happens if the city council does not accept the report? Would the mayor drop her initiative?"

Dawson answered, "No. The mayor is committed to promoting sustainability; she is fully behind the report."

Smith added, "I understand that councilman Brown is writing a resolution that will specify that a vote to accept the report is not an endorsement of it. Would that be acceptable to you?"

Odell and Dawson echoed each other in quickly replying that it would be. Then Dawson explained that in the legislature acceptance of a report does not mean endorsement of it. "In Olympia we frequently accepted reports that we did not entirely endorse. It was a way of appreciating the work of the people who put the report together for us."

At that point, Professor England had had enough. "I have to say that I, personally, would not be happy if the council accepted the report in that fashion. The report is not simply a statement of findings. At its heart, it is a set of recommendations. If the city council's acceptance simply means that they have received it and appreciate all of our hard work, the recommendations could easily be ignored. They do not have to accept all of the specific recommendations, but they should accept them in principle, agree to move in the direction of the recommendations, and agree to further study them to see which ones they want to have implemented."

Knudtson quickly interjected, "But that is not for us to decide. The council can decide what they *mean* by accepting the report. We just hope that they *will* accept it. If Brown's resolution is the way they accept it, we probably have at least a 4 to 3 majority."

Porter changed the topic. "So, what were you wanting to talk to us about?"

Dawson took the lead. "We were hoping that the board would be interested in writing an editorial in support of the task force report. Because of their colorfully exaggerated (and wrong) statements, the anti-global warming people

206   LARRY S. LUTON

have been getting more attention than we think they deserve. An editorial in support of the task force report would do something to counteract that.

"The report is the result of a local, community-based effort. Hundreds of people offered nearly a thousand suggestions. The meetings were open and inclusive. The report is a menu of possible solutions for the city to consider. It recommends incentives. It does not include mandates.

"As I think you know, the recommendations in the report would be worth following whether or not we were facing global warming. The central tenets are stewardship and efficiency. They make economic sense. They are fiscally responsible and would save money in the long run. Sustainability is a good principle to follow. It will make the city more resilient, no matter what the future holds."

Porter reminded the task force members that editorial positions were the collective position of the board and said he would see what the board wanted to do.

A couple of days later, Smith addressed the topic in his "Sharp Points" column, critiquing the claims of the opposition and supporting the task force recommendations as sensible steps for the city to take.

* * *

Sunday afternoon, prior to the Monday evening meeting at which the city council was expected to vote on the task force plan, Jason and Courtney walked to The Grind and Knead, a neighborhood bakery and coffee shop, just to sit at a table, enjoy the day, and talk with each other. They often did this and found that their conversations roamed freely over a wide variety of the aspects of their lives. This day it was no surprise that their conversation quickly turned to a discussion of his experience with the task force and his sense of what the city council might do.

It was actually Courtney who brought up the subject. "Well, Jason, tomorrow's the big day. How are you feeling about what will happen at the city council meeting?"

"It looks to me like a resolution to 'accept' the plan will pass, but that may not be as good as sounds. Councilman Brown is working on a resolution that will make it clear that accepting the report does not mean that the council agrees to do what it recommends."

"What about the bigger picture? Has this work on the task force been a good experience?"

"It's a mixed bag. I've learned a lot about organizational change and citizen participation in governance, but what I've learned is not necessarily encouraging. Organizational change is more difficult than I realized. It takes time, patience, and a significant commitment from the leaders to make it happen. I know the mayor believes in sustainability, but I am not sure she put enough into this effort. Trying to make this kind of change in one year was probably asking too much. That deadline was imposed by the economic development grant, but the grant did not provide enough resources to really make things happen. I'm not sure it was worth the money to place the whole time frame of the task force within its limits.

"Citizen participation is an appropriate ideal for a democracy, but it too takes a lot more time and effort than I realized to be done well. You have to match the level of energy and commitment you can reasonably expect from citizens to the role you have them play in the process. Some of them simply want to be heard. Others want varying degrees of decision-making authority— sometimes more than they can have. Interest groups think they represent the wishes of the citizens, but they are not authorized representatives like the elected officials. The elected officials are the ones who have gone through a democratic process and are, therefore, authorized to make decisions based on their views of what the people want or need. Still, sometimes it is difficult to see them as much more representative than the interest groups.

"On the other hand, this experience will help me be more prepared for similar challenges in the future. I am sure that this is not the last time I will be involved in trying to overcome organizational inertia or involving citizens in meaningful participation in decisions that affect their lives."

Changing the subject, Courtney asked, "How do you think this will impact your career? When this all started, you said it was an opportunity to move your career forward."

"I'm not sure. It may be that the connections I made and the opportunities I had to show what kind of work I can do will be the keys to progress on that front. I feel confident that I made a good impression on the mayor and Wellsworth—and the rest of the task force. I'm not so sure about the city department heads. I don't think the city council even connects me to the task force report, which in some ways is disappointing, but given their take on the action plan may not be bad."

* * *

When the city council began taking testimony at its next meeting about the task force report, council president Sweeney admonished those speaking not to be redundant and asked those who spoke at the last meeting to allow new people to speak first. Finally, he reminded them to keep their comments short.

The first speaker that night said, "The problem I have with this sustainability thing is the origins of it. It goes back to the Kyoto Treaty, UN Agenda 21,

208   LARRY S. LUTON

and the Brudtland Commission report, which was written by a socialist from Norway. It's about communitarianism and against everything that America stands for. The mayor does not have the authority to sign an international treaty—which is what this is. Do not limit the rights of citizens."

The next opponent suggested that the last thing needed with the economy in the hole was to adopt more regulations and higher taxes. Others suggested that the sustainability report promoted electric cars and, therefore, would reward the wealthy. One argued that global warming was based on faulty science and that we were actually entering a new ice age. He said that "Global warming is a blatant lie put forth in the media." Another complained that she did not want her children to become "faucet police." Yet another said that he did not hate nature, but the report set down environmental goals as absolute requirements. "The purpose of government is not to protect the environment from the citizens. You need to reject this new green religion of sustainability. Please put this green genie back in the bottle before it's too late."

The first supporter of the sustainability report told the council, "This is not a treaty. It is about our local community taking control of our local environment. Let's look at this report a different way. What if we flipped the recommendations and looked at their opposites? Do we want to *not* improve continuously? Should we promote *dirty* mobility? *Not* enable optimal land use? *Not* conserve water? *Not* prepare through planning? Not doing these things makes no sense."

Another supporter suggested that the recommendations would help the community compete with cities like Portland and Seattle, and that their options would only become more limited the longer they delayed adopting sustainability. He also pointed out that cost-benefit analysis would take place before anything was done.

A third reminded the council that the United States was at the origin of the environmental movement, which was led by such people as Teddy Roosevelt, John Muir, Aldo Leopold, and William Douglas. "Environmentalism is as American as apple pie. In adopting this plan the city will be acting in the best American tradition and be leading by example, not telling others what to do."

Having waited for all the new people to make their comments, the Tea Party member, Polson, returned to the podium to warn the council. "This report may look simple and straightforward. It may sound good, but there are lots of hidden agendas in it. There are all kinds of blowback on things that sound good. It is a plan that the city cannot sustain."

The former state senator, Adams, also returned to make a final comment. "Do you have a fiscal note? This report would put a real burden on small businesses—mandates, regulations, costs. With the economy in a mess, this

THINK GLOBAL, ACT LOCAL? 209

is not the time to add more layers of government, more taxes, more fees. It is a kind of cannibalism on the existing system. It is a foreign agenda in our country. If someone outside the country is visiting their policies on us, that is a frightening situation. It means our government is not in control."

Recognizing that the testimony from the public had concluded, Mayor Lightfoot made her way to the podium. "Many of the comments you have heard tonight and last week come from an ideological bent that really has almost nothing to do with what has been presented to you. This report is composed of locally driven ideas. It is based on common sense and the principle of good stewardship.

"I eagerly seek your action on this report. The sustainability task force report is not something for you to reluctantly accept, but for you to eagerly embrace. Those who would have you reject it may have good intentions, but they have bad information. They have presented trumped-up speculation that is completely refuted by the record. Do not let a small group of citizens with a shrill misinformation campaign keep you from doing the right thing.

"The process that resulted in the sustainability report was thorough and broad-based. It will save real money in real time without a single mandate."

Then the council began its deliberations.

Harrison in his workshirt blue dress shirt and with his identification tag lanyard dangling from around his neck, talked about how the world has or will soon reach the point of "peak oil." After that point less oil will be discovered and it will cost much more to retrieve. "We will be in a situation of increasing demand and decreasing supply. I wholeheartedly support this plan."

Sporting a dark navy blue blazer and a navy tie with yellow polka dots, the tall, gray-haired council member Walker spoke next. "We receive all kinds of reports and plans. We do not need to agree with every aspect. The council must approve any expenditures. All we're being asked to do is accept the recommendations and keep them in mind as we act in the future. A bad economy requires greater stewardship. I want to see a positive message that these principles are important."

Pearson rolled up the sleeves of his shirt and replied, "An action plan requires that we all get behind it. The opposition to this plan isn't just a handful of people." Waving his hands, he continued, "This is more divisive than any plan I've ever seen here. Besides, we are already being good stewards of the public resources. I could go on all night about the things we are already doing. I can't support this, not because it's not good, but because the public can't grasp it."

His flag pin prominent on the lapel of his charcoal gray three-piece suit, Brown entered the discussion to offer his motion. "I want to say thank you to the committee and to the opposition to it. You have all worked hard to make this discussion a fine example of democracy at work.

"I move that the city council accept the mayor's task force action plan. By accepting the plan, the city council acknowledges receipt of the plan and its recommendations. Acceptance of the plan does not constitute final legislative action by the city council to adopt or implement the plan or its recommendations. Any further actions relating to the recommendations contained in the plan shall only occur after a thorough financial analysis and feasibility study on the merits of specific recommendations. The city council as the legislative body shall review the results of the analyses and studies and, where appropriate, take subsequent legislative action, after public input and council deliberation, to adopt the appropriate ordinance, resolution, or other legislative action."

Wearing a burnt orange open-collar silk shirt with the sleeves neatly folded halfway up to his elbows, Lockwood leaned forward to peer over his glasses and spoke next. "I want to thank Councilman Brown for making his motion. In our meetings on this plan, both sides showed great passion. It is not only what you do, but why you do it. If the environmental aspects of this are disturbing, take them out and you still have good policy statements for the city to follow. I did not like the aspect of this that was an action plan. 'Green jobs' can mean many things. We need to be careful."

Sweeney brusquely joined in. "There is widespread agreement on the fact of global warming—maybe not on the causes. In accepting this report, we are not going to be adopting any political philosophies. All we are doing is acknowledging that we got the report."

Edwards put on a big smile like an elementary schoolteacher who was about to explain a new rule to her class and eased into her opposition to the report. "There are parts of this plan I could support, but here are my issues. The action plan is based on three items: climate mitigation, climate adaptation, and energy security.

"We don't want to limit our sources of energy. Let the market determine what energy we use.

"There is no consensus on the science. We should be concerned about global cooling. Predictions of global warming are based on climate models and we all know the frailty of models. It is not carbon dioxide that controls the climate but water vapor. As Dr. Richard Lindzen of MIT has said, the apparent scientific consensus on global warming is the product of *pressures* on the scientific community to participate in 'climate alarmism.'

"We are living in a fiscally disturbing time. Once our finances are in order, then we can move on to other concerns. We need *fiscal* sustainability first."

Pearson joined in. "Councilman Brown's motion amends the sustainability

THINK GLOBAL, ACT LOCAL? 211

action plan into a simple report, but I still can't support it—because it's nothing! As an action plan, it is divisive. As a report, it does nothing. I'm sorry, but that's the way I see it."

Walker countered with a slight edge in his voice. "When we accept a plan, it does not constitute final authority or obligate financial expenditures, but when I vote to accept it, it's an endorsement, an indication of support of the principles."

Harrison offered a simple final comment. "Adoption of the plan is prudent and conservative and fiscally responsible."

Sweeney looked to each councilmember and asked if there were any further comments. Hearing none, he called for the vote.

The electronic board showed the vote:

> Brown—Yes
> Edwards—No
> Harrison—Yes
> Lockwood—Yes
> Pearson—No
> Sweeney—Yes
> Walker—Yes

Sweeney announced the tally: "The motion passes, five to two. There being no further business, we are adjourned."

* * *

Later that evening, Jason and Courtney sat in their living room with a glass of wine and discussed what had happened at the council meeting.

"So you won!" Courtney opined.

"I'm not so sure," said Jason. "For me, the motion by Brown took away the victory."

"But you got a 5–2 vote. Isn't that a win? Won't the mayor be happy with that?"

"Yeah, she'll certainly describe it as a win. For her, 'acceptance' is what will matter. Not the content of the motion. But Brown's motion said that acceptance of the plan simply meant that they had received it, not that they endorsed it. But even if there had been no motion, their acceptance of the plan would not have led directly to action. The council would have had to support and fund specific actions. The motion's real impact was to signal their lack of support. I think that means that they will never act on implementing it. Nothing will change."

"Will the mayor be able to implement parts of it without further council action? Doesn't she have authority to get city departments to make changes? She is the chief executive, isn't she?"

"She will be able to keep the Green Team alive, and they will discuss things the departments can do to promote sustainability. They may even be able to get their departments to make small changes, but without the city council pushing, the departments will probably continue to operate as they always have. Many people in the departments were less than excited about the sustainability initiative. They'll know how empty the vote was and feel safe in dragging their feet. There is no political will to keep it going."

"That's too bad, honey, but we do live in a pretty conservative town. Maybe that is an accurate reflection of the will of the people."

* * *

Early the next day, Rebecca Polson sent an e-mail to Rush Limbaugh that began, "As a member of our local Tea Party, I am sad to report that last night the jackbooted, greenshirt, enviro-Nazis won a major victory in our city council. . . ."

Part IV
Imaging the Possibilities

The final chapter brings together the themes and discusses the potential for collaboration and co-creation with citizens and the kinds of radical, positive change in behaviors and institutions that are possible.

13

Imagining the Possibilities

Cheryl Simrell King and Ryan K. Warner

The individual chapters of this edited volume come together to tell a compelling story about the relationships, and the possibilities, amongst and between citizens and their governments. The story is about the possibilities of governing differently, in ways that don't oppress, marginalize, or limit people, and about bringing different sensibilities to the practices of administration. The Progressive era administrator—one who is the expert, is "in charge," and, through the proper management tools, will administer the "right" way—is an administrator of the past. The Progressive era administrator's habit of mind emphasized managerial control over administrative processes. This administrative stance is doomed in situations in which difference and disagreement bring us to the table instead of agreement and similarities, and in situations where we are least likely to work together because of political, ideological, racial, ethnic, economic, and social differences. In a word, Progressive era administration cannot serve us in contemporary times. True, we can make the trains run on time, but everything else about train operation can be subjected to different interpretations, depending upon where the interpreters stand.

In the first edition of this book we called for "active administration," which moved past hierarchical and elitist views of administration and toward a more horizontal, shared authority, or what Terry Cooper (1991, 140) calls "power with." Active administration was not an enhancement of administrative power, but the use of discretionary authority to foster and facilitate collaborative work with citizens. A horizontal administrator is more collaborative, relying on citizens and other stakeholders for guidance and acting as a facilitator of processes and institutions. Now, while we would still argue for active administration, fifteen years of research and practice tell us that facilitation of processes is not enough to positively affect relationships amongst and between citizens and their governments.

Facilitative Leadership

John Forester (2010), in his most recent work, expands the job of a citizen-centered administrator beyond that of facilitator. In order to make public participation and democratic deliberation work in an environment where our differences are more likely to bring us together to the table rather than our similarities, contemporary administrators need to *facilitate, moderate,* and *mediate* action, in what he calls facilitative leadership. Forester says:

> To promote a dialogue, we must *facilitate* conversations; to promote a debate, we must *moderate* an argument; to *promote* a successful negotiation, we must *mediate* proposals for action. (5)

According to Forester, "facilitative leaders" work to "enable well-informed decisions by parties so they may level the playing field of preexisting inequalities of information and access to relative expertise" (4–5).

The themes that emerge out of the chapters in this book go hand-in-hand with Forester's vision of administrators who approach the realities of public situations with eyes wide open to the dilemmas and possibilities of their work, recognizing that facilitating and mediating collaborative action means moving beyond idealism about citizen engagement and participation to practices that can harness both positive and negative participatory energy.

Democratic Action

Democratic action can happen anywhere and should happen in places other than politics and administration, or it is not likely to be a strong force. Where it happens is extremely important, as Rawlings and Catlaw argue in their call to think about democracy as something bigger than what public administrators facilitate in their work. Conversely, where it happens is also not important; that is, it can happen in nonprofits and other organizations doing public work and still potentially have a positive affect on citizenship and the relationships between citizens and governments.

Represent Our Citizens

As facilitators and moderators of processes and mediators of action, we can bring citizen sensibilities to the table, even if citizens are not represented. We can imagine citizens' lives and bring that information to the table, as Box says, and following on Hannah Arendt's notion of "visiting" where we imagine things we don't know. We can also imagine alternative futures, thinking be-

Box 13.1
A Few Words from Joseph Gray

Joseph Gray, along with his coauthor Linda Chapin, wrote the final chapter of the first edition of this book. Their chapter served as the culminating words as they described a very successful citizen-centered process in Orange County, Florida—Targeted Community Initiative—which was the embodiment of what the contributors to the first edition recommended. Gray left the job with Orange County after a newly elected county executive disbanded the initiative. Joe has been doing citizen-centered planning and development since then, as a private consultant and, when necessary, as a local government employee.

I guess my perspective today is about the same as it was when Linda Chapin and I wrote that chapter. It was an aspiration and my aspirations haven't changed. My work has, however, made me a bit more pessimistic.

I'm basically doing the same work right now, just in different ways. I'm currently focused on developing community land trusts for affordable housing and commercial development. To me, it's the ultimate form of participatory governance and the ultimate opportunity for citizen-government partnerships. At center is something that is at the core of America—owning land and property—and creating opportunities for impoverished communities to gain wealth. We do two things: (1) create opportunities for personal wealth building and home ownership on an individual level; and (2) create opportunities for collective community ownership of neighborhoods and control of those assets. This is an opportunity for folks in distressed neighborhoods to control their destiny as well as be involved in the management of their endeavors.

One of basic tenets of a "classic" community land trust (CLT) is a tripartite governance structure: one-third are people who live in CLT housing, one-third are neighbors, one-third are business interests/stakeholders. However, the governance role resides in the background—it's mostly about making sure the assets are stewarded in a responsible manner. People who serve in the governance structures are much more likely to engage in other community-based activities. They end up on other boards and develop confidence and skills.

For example, I'm working with the Ford Foundation on setting up land trusts in New Orleans (lower Ninth Ward). Ford Foundation's lament is that they spent the last twenty-five years supporting community development corporations (CDCs), but most CDCs haven't been much of a force in terms of working with communities beyond simply qualifying home buyers. After the first purchase, the homes are turned over to the market. This doesn't happen in land trusts—the homes become part of the trust and remain per-

(continued)

manently affordable. The trust is about sustaining the community through physical revitalization, education, and financial literacy. As a result, the communities are much better prepared to be codesigners of their solutions and coproducers of actions. The playing field is leveled.

Most land is donated by governments. The other area where governments play a huge role is in subsidies (community development block grant funds—HOME Investment Partnership program dollars). For the last fifty years or so, the federal government has been giving that money away to individuals—after the original beneficiary sells that house, they are back to square one. More and more, governments are starting to sponsor and create their own land trusts, which is somewhat troubling. When governments are at the center, you start to lose the "c" in community land trusts. Community gets squeezed out, and these should be community projects. The appropriate role of government is to enable citizens and to direct funds toward the common good.

Here's what I have to say to people interested in improving citizen-government relationships: Citizens, more than ever, have to take responsibility to go beyond sound bites about government and get involved at the local level, where the action is. If we don't do it, I'm afraid of where we are headed, in terms of our country and its entire governance structure. As long as we just keep seeing government as something other than us, it's easy for us to hate it. Until we start to realize that the only way we are going to control this thing is by us taking the time to understand all those issues that we are just passing off on government—until we start taking responsibility at community level—not much us going to change. So, we are back to the basics: educating and organizing. And it should be easier than ever to do this with the Internet and through social media. As more and more people become connected, we should take advantage to do more than connect socially, the technology can be a powerful force for bringing people together. We see examples of it in developing countries all over the world, where people are organizing and being positive forces in governance.

To government workers I say we have to keep preaching the gospel, now more than ever. You have to show people things nowadays—you have to take some action, have meaningful outcomes. That's why I like working with community land trusts—we can clearly and quickly demonstrate people coming together and taking control of their community and people can see the differences they are making. We need to make opportunities to participate in real ways, not just in dialogue but in action. We have to have results, not just from an accountability perspective but because action and meaningful results are what keep people working and at the table. It's all about building houses and building neighborhoods—period. The process is almost irrelevant, other than having the right people there. It's really about outcomes.

IMAGINING THE POSSIBILITIES   219

yond present circumstances to consciously shape, or design, future conditions rather than waiting for them to happen. And, as Kovalick, Walts, and Wells tell us, it is essential to level the playing field and bring a sense of "curiosity" to one's work with citizens.

Level the Playing Field

To state it again: leveling the playing field is key—people around the table need to have equal footing. One way to level the playing field is through information sharing and education. We can take a stance toward this work that, as Forester says:

> . . . stresses public learning, recognizing differences of interests, values, and power, the power of asking good question, and always anticipating structured biases related to ethnicity and culture, race, class, gender and more. (15–16)

Collaboration

As facilitators and moderators of processes and mediators of action we don't discount the role of the administrator at the table; collaborative work is not turning over all power and authority to citizens; it is about working together. As Timney says, collaboration may help to change perceptions of administrators as the enemy and recognizes that administrators have value in decision processes.

Improve Relationships

Improving relationships requires that we, as administrators, bring a different "I" or "us" to the table. More important, perhaps, than knowing how to use Excel to make a budget, are skills in mediation, facilitation, moderation, and dealing with difference. And, perhaps more important than managerial values are those values that allow us to practice acts of reciprocal kindness; our relationships with citizens are reciprocal relationships. A good sense of ourselves is very important, as is a level of self-reflectivity that will allow us to weather very difficult conversations with people who do agree with each other or with us, conversations that can get uncivil. Does this mean we should rethink what we are doing in educating administrators? Does this mean we should be using different variables in hiring decisions?

Technology

Conversations about citizen-government relationships need to include a discussion about technology. Social media and other technological innovations have changed the landscape of networking and communicating. The legal questions about government use of social media sites are still unanswered. Still, it is very important to consider these methods because of generational differences in their use. The so-called dutifuls (those born before 1945) and the baby boomers (born 1946–64) are rapidly aging, and Gen Xers (1965–76) and individuals born after 1976 (Generation Y) have very different relationships with social media than their older counterparts. The presumption that experience equals the knowledge we no longer need holds true. Boomers, who hold the majority of leadership positions in administration, may not only lack the knowledge needed, we also don't know what questions to ask. This is not just about learning how to use a new tool—we need to learn a new way of being in the world. It may be time for boomers to get out of the way and open up leadership, whether positional or not, to those who have the skills and perspectives needed to administer in these complex contexts. At the very least, we have to start listening to those in other generations and to appreciate that a participatory awakening of these new generations requires overcoming decades of forces that have worked to push them against traditional politics and participation (Zukin et al. 2006). The Obama campaign's use of the Internet and social media methods to capture these two generations is illustrative of the power of these new approaches to participation and engagement. The leveling of satisfaction with his presidency and the concomitant political disengagement of these generations speaks to the importance of linking results with new methods of engagement. As Joseph Gray tells us, action—results—are what matter.

Participation Methods

We need to develop and adopt participation methods that consider diversity. Very little is known about cultural differences in participation; we need to know more. All techniques do not apply universally and the techniques that work most for the privileged (those who in the past were most likely to participate) may not work for others.

Working Together

We can't get very far with citizen engagement efforts if we are oppressing or marginalizing others, whether by our behavior or institutional norms. Improving relationships amongst and between citizens and governments has to start with cleaning house, so to speak, within our organizations and within ourselves, as illustrated in the stories about Seattle's Race and Social Justice Initiative (Chapter 10) and the City of Olympia (Chapter 11). Kwame Anthony

IMAGING THE POSSIBILITIES   221

Appiah (2006) calls upon us to engage in conversations, "in particular, conversation between people from different ways of life" (xxi). He continues:

> The problem of cross-cultural communication can seem immensely difficult in theory when we are trying to imagine making sense of a stranger in the abstract. But the great lesson of anthropology is that when the stranger is no longer imaginary, but real and present, sharing a human social life, you may like or dislike him, you may agree or disagree, but, if it is what you both want, you can make some sense of each other in the end. (99)

Organizational Change

While our personal practices and behaviors are important, if we don't make the concomitant organizational and institutional changes, we aren't going to get very far. And we need to be politically savvy and ready to have things happen that are beyond our control. The way down the path to organizational and institutional change involves two steps forward and one step back. And organizational culture change takes many years to come to fruition.

Portals and Movements

Problematic relationships can be approached through a series of portals. One can be organizational change, as the Seattle case shows us. Other openings or portals, such as sustainability and environmental justice, can also serve the same ends, but one should heed the cautionary tale of Luton's fictional character, Jason Allen. Sometimes one can be merely a pawn in a bigger game, leading to inauthentic efforts that further frustrate citizens and administrators.

In short, we need to be different kinds of administrators than we have been in the past and recognize that citizens are not all the same. The same techniques don't work for all people, and we are just beginning to understand cultural differences in participation and engagement. Although government may be us, that "Us" is not monolingual or monocultural. Each person comes to the public table with a different picture of what participation looks like and what their role could be. One group may best communicate their needs and opinions through an online survey, chat group, or other electronic medium. Another group may more easily share their lived experience through a public meeting at a local town hall, community center, or diner. As an example, when transportation planners in Washington State attempted to solicit feedback from special needs transportation users[1] about their requirements for a public bus system, planners found their outreach most successful when they personally targeted and invited each group to provide feedback. The feedback they received from seniors was very different than the information they received from teens, just as access to the system for people with disabilities and poor was different from access to the system for others. If not identified and specifically targeted, many of these groups would likely have been left out of the process.

While we say that this book is a bit more sober, pragmatic, and realistic than the first edition of *Government Is Us,* the contributors to this text agree that government can be us, if it isn't now. We also agree, for the most part, that government can be significantly improved if more views are represented and if we are better able to bring different, disagreeing voices together and work to mediate successful proposals for action, in the spirit of Forester (2010). As stated earlier, we are not offering citizen engagement as a panacea for all that ails us. What we hope to have offered are some ideas and examples of changes that can be made to make our governance institutions more participatory and socially just, as well as to make our government more "us," a goal that was innovative and laudable at the birth of this nation and has remained so throughout our history. This text does not put this goal to rest: we will always need to revise and revitalize our work to ensure our governments and administrations are participatory and just and that government is "us." We hope this work continues with you, the reader, and with those you interact and co-govern with throughout your work in public service.

Note

1. Defined in Washington State Law as those who because of age, income, or disability cannot access transportation.

References

Appiah, Kwame Anthony. 2006. *Cosmopolitanism: Ethics in a World of Strangers.* New York: Norton & Company.
Cooper, Terry L. 1991. *An Ethic of Citizenship for Public Administration.* Englewood Cliffs, NJ: Prentice Hall.
Forester, John. 2010. *Dealing with Differences: Dramas of Mediating Public Disputes.* New York: Oxford University Press.
Zukin, Cliff, Scott Keeter, Molly Andolina, Krista Jenkins, and Michael X. Delli Carpini. 2006. *A New Engagement: Political Participation, Civic Life, and the Changing American Citizen.* New York: Oxford University Press.

About the Editor and Contributors

Jennifer K. Alexander is director of the Master of Public Administration and the Master of Nonprofit Administration and Leadership degree programs at the Maxine Goodman Levin College of Urban Affairs at Cleveland State University and Co-Director of the Center for Nonprofit Policy and Practice. Her research includes civil society, administrative responsibility, and public-nonprofit partnerships. Dr. Alexander received her PhD from the Center for Public Administration and Policy at Virginia Tech and a bachelor of science degree in foreign service from Georgetown University.

Richard C. Box is Regents/Foundation professor in the School of Public Administration, University of Nebraska at Omaha. His writing focuses on the role of the public service practitioner in a democratic society and the application of critical theory in public administration. He is the author or editor of *Citizen Governance: Leading American Communities into the 21st Century* (Sage Publications, 1998); *Public Administration and Society: Critical Issues in American Governance* (M.E. Sharpe, 2004; 2d ed., 2009); *Critical Social Theory in Public Administration* (M.E. Sharpe, 2005); *Democracy and Public Administration* (M.E. Sharpe, 2007); and *Making a Difference: Progressive Values in Public Administration* (M.E. Sharpe, 2008).

Elliott Bronstein is the public information officer for the City of Seattle's Office for Civil Rights (SOCR), and serves on the Race and Social Justice Initiative's coordinating committee. Prior to joining SOCR, Mr. Bronstein served for fifteen years as the editor of *The Voice,* a monthly newspaper for public housing residents in Seattle-King County. He hails from Winnipeg Manitoba, Canada. He is the father of two daughters.

224 ABOUT THE EDITOR AND CONTRIBUTORS

Thomas J. Catlaw is associate professor in the School of Public Affairs at Arizona State University in Phoenix. His research centers on the application of psychoanalytic and postmodern theory to problems of governance, authority, legitimacy, and political change. His work has appeared in *American Behavioral Scientist, Administration & Society, Administrative Theory & Praxis, Public Administration Review,* and the *American Review of Public Administration,* among other venues. His first book, *Fabricating the People: Politics and Administration in the Biopolitical State,* was published by the University of Alabama Press in 2007. Dr. Catlaw is also the current editor of *Administrative Theory & Praxis,* an international journal dedicated to the theoretical and critical analysis of governmental practice. He worked previously for the U.S. Office of Management and Budget in the Executive Office of the President, and the Center for Excellence in Municipal Management in Washington, DC.

Glenn Harris is the manager of the Race and Social Justice Initiative. He previously served four years with the City of Seattle's Department of Neighborhoods as the Coordinator for the Southeast District, one of the most diverse neighborhoods in the United States. Mr. Harris came to city government after four years as development director and antiracism trainer with Western States Center, a Portland-based nonprofit that provides technical assistance, training, and policy analysis to social change organizations.

Ron Harris-White is special projects manager in the office of the Seattle Parks and Recreation Superintendent and serves as the executive sponsor for the department's Race and Social Justice Change Team. He has more than twenty years experience in community involvement and public administration, and has been involved with the Race and Social Justice Initiative since its inception. Mr. Harris-White holds two master's degrees and currently co-chairs the King County Food and Fitness Initiative.

Cheryl Simrell King is a member of the faculty at The Evergreen State College, teaching primarily in the Master of Public Administration (MPA) Program. She is coauthor of *Transformative Public Service: Portraits of Theory in Practice* (M.E. Sharpe, 2005) and *Government Is Us: Public Administration in an Anti-Government Era* (Sage, 1998), as well as articles in other trade press and academic journals. She writes and practices in the areas of democratizing and transforming public administration, accountability, sustainability, and the relationships amongst and between citizens and their governments. Dr. King's current public service work focuses on transformational local government sustainability initiatives and assisting local government officials in designing and implementing citizen engagement endeavors.

Walter W. Kovalick Jr. acts as the senior official for management and administration for the U.S. Environmental Protection Agency's regional office in Chicago. For this 1,200-person organization, his responsibilities encompass human resources, information technology, geographic information support, facilities, budget, contracts and grants, and the regional laboratory. As a charter member of the EPA, his program experience includes the air, hazardous waste, toxic substances, Superfund, and innovative technology (for site cleanup) programs. He worked on the design and implementation of public involvement efforts related to the EPA's chemical regulatory and Superfund programs. He has served on advisory committees of the National Research Council and the Department of Energy and has been a consultant to the German government, the city of Sao Paulo, the United Nations Environment Program, and the World Bank Global Environment Facility. He has chaired several multinational pilot studies under the auspices of the NATO Science for Peace and Security programs.

Larry S. Luton is a professor of public administration and directs the MPA Program at Eastern Washington University, where he has worked for more than twenty-five years. His research interests include research approaches in public administration, environmental policy administration, public administration history, and administrative law. He has had articles published in a number of journals, including *Administration & Society, Public Administration Review, Policy Studies Journal,* and *Administrative Theory & Praxis.* His first book was *The Politics of Garbage* (University of Pittsburgh Press, 1996), and his most recent book is *Qualitative Research Approaches for Public Administration* (M.E. Sharpe, 2010).

Claire Mostel recently retired from Miami-Dade County after eighteen years of service. She served as outreach supervisor for Team Metro for thirteen years and compliance support coordinator for the office of neighborhood compliance for one year. Prior to working for Team Metro, she served as the clerk of courts for four years. Claire joined Miami-Dade County after working at Florida International University. She is an adjunct professor at Barry University and received her bachelor's and master's degrees in public administration from Florida International University.

Michael Mucha has been a leader in city government for twenty years, with appointments in Wisconsin, Pennsylvania, and Washington. He most recently was the director of public works for the City of Olympia and currently serves as chief engineer and director of the Madison (Wisconsin)

226 ABOUT THE EDITOR AND CONTRIBUTORS

Metropolitan Sewerage District. He received his bachelor's of science degree in civil engineering from the University of Wisconsin and his master's in public administration from the University of Washington. He also completed Harvard's Senior Executives program. Mr. Mucha is a registered professional engineer in three states.

Renee Nank is an assistant professor of public administration at the University of Texas San Antonio. Professor Nank's current research foci include intersectoral relationships between the public and nonprofit sectors, disaster resiliency, and civil society organizations in Mexico.

Julie Nelson is the director of the Seattle Office for Civil Rights, which coordinates the Race and Social Justice Initiative. She has worked for the City of Seattle since 1988, with technical and management experience in the Human Services, City Light, Public Utilities, and Executive Administration departments. She received her bachelor of arts degree from the University of Arizona and her master's degree in economics from the University of Washington. Ms. Nelson is the mother of two teenage boys.

Kelly Campbell Rawlings is an assistant professor in the department of politics and international affairs at Northern Arizona University. Her research focuses on the intersections between civic engagement, democratic governance, and civil society as well as the development of civic capacity and transformational leadership. Her work has been published in *Administration & Society* and the *Journal of Public Affairs Education* (as Kelly B. Campbell). Prior to academia, Dr. Rawlings worked in the nonprofit sector as a prevention education specialist for the Center Against Sexual Abuse and as a policy advocate for the Arizona Coalition Against Domestic Violence. She has also worked as an academic associate for Arizona State University's Lodestar Center for Philanthropy and Nonprofit Innovation, where she conducted research on the nonprofit sector and developed and coordinated projects designed to build the organizational capacity of the nonprofit sector.

Mary M. Timney, PhD, is professor of public administration at Pace University in New York. Her teaching responsibilities include administrative ethics, organization theory, and primary adviser for the capstone project. She created the course in citizen participation and is developing a new course in sustainable management for public administrators. Dr. Timney's interest in citizen participation began when she was an environmental activist in the early 1970s and served as executive director of the Allegheny County Environmental Coalition in Pittsburgh. Dr. Timney's research interests include energy and environmental policy, citizen participation, and public administration theory. Her articles have been published in *Public Administration Review, Administrative Theory & Praxis,* and *Public Productivity Review.* Her recent book, *Power for the People,* examines the impacts of electricity deregulation on state energy policy using the California experience as a case study. It is also a critique on using the market to achieve public policy goals. She has presented numerous papers over the past twenty-six years at conferences such as the American Society for Public Administration, the Public Administration Theory Network, and the American Political Science Association.

Alan Walts is director of the Office of Enforcement and Compliance Assurance for U.S. EPA Region 5. He received his Juris Doctorate from University of Michigan Law School in 1995, and started as legal counsel for EPA Region 5 in 1996.

Ryan K. Warner has an extensive background in public service and over the past fifteen years has focused his talents on human rights, the law, and improving the lives of people with disabilities. He is currently the special needs planner at the Washington State Department of Transportation focusing on Accessibility and Coordinated Transportation. Ryan received his bachelor of arts degree from The Evergreen State College in 1996 and his master of public administration in 2006. He lives in Olympia, Washington, with his wife and two-and-a-half-year-old son. When not working he enjoys reading, enjoying the wonders of nature in the Pacific Northwest, and spending time with family and friends.

Suzanne Wells is director of the Superfund Community Involvement and Program Initiatives Branch in the Office of Superfund Remediation and Technology Innovation at the U.S. Environmental Protection Agency. Ms. Wells has worked at the EPA since 1983 and with the Superfund program since 1987. In addition to directing the national Superfund community involvement program, she has served as acting deputy director of the Superfund Office of Program Management, was responsible for implementation of revisions to the Hazard Ranking System and development of eligibility policies for placing contaminated sites on the National Priorities List, and co-chaired development of the Superfund Green Remediation Strategy. In 2007, Ms. Wells was a Brookings Institution LEGIS/Congressional Fellow and worked for Senator Ken Salazar. She has a bachelor of science degree in Environmental Science from Texas Christian University, and a master's degree in Technology and Human Affairs from Washington University. She also holds a Conflict Management Certificate from the USDA Graduate School.

228 ABOUT THE EDITOR AND CONTRIBUTORS

Lisa A. Zanetti is an associate professor in the Harry S. Truman School of Public Affairs at the University of Missouri. She was a collaborator on *Government Is Us: Public Administration in an Anti-Government Age* (Sage, 1998) and coauthor with Cheryl Simrell King of *Transformational Public Service: Portraits of Theory in Practice* (M.E. Sharpe, 2005). She is currently working on a book about empathy in disaster situations. Her articles have appeared in *Administrative Theory & Praxis, American Review of Public Administration, Administration & Society, Human Relations, Tamara, Journal of Organizational Change Management,* and other outlets. She remains cancer free.

Index

Accountability
citizen discontent, 12, 13, 18–19
nonprofit partnerships, 101, 112
Active administration, 215
Active citizenship
citizen discontent, 6, 13–14
nonprofit partnerships, 102–3, 105
Active participation model
model characteristics, 91 (table)
model expansion, 86, 93 (table)
Addams, Jane, 64
Affective empathy, 83
AIDS patients, 78–79
American Dream, 8, 42
American Federation of State, County,
and Municipal Employees
(AFSCME), 181
American Society for Public
Administration, Code of Ethics, 83
America*Speaks*
Internet Web site, 24, 95
"Listen to the City" (New York), 24,
95, 96–97
Washington, DC, Citizen Summits,
95–96
Anderson, Leif, 168
Annie E. Casey Foundation, 103
Anti-global warming activists, 201,
203, 204, 205–6, 207–12

Antigovernment movements, 5, 13
Arnstein, S., 17
Astroturf-roots politics, 87
Athenian democracy model, 63–64
Audacity of Hope, The (Obama), 78
Avino, Joaquin, 148

Boat People SOS, 127
Brady, H., 39
Budget and Policy Filter (Seattle,
Washington), 169
Bureaucrats, 5
Bureau Men, Settlement Women
(Stivers), 107
Bush, George H.W., 130
Business group engagement
contracting services, 163–65, 169–70
environmental sustainability
narrative, 188, 189, 193, 197–99,
200, 204–6
historically underutilized businesses
(HUB), 163–65
women and minority business
enterprises (WMBE), 163–64

Cabrillo Marine Aquarium, 127
California
environmental permits, 126
Palos Verdes Shelf, 127

230 INDEX

California *(continued)*
  Proposition 13, 7
  Proposition 209, 164
Capacity building, 160, 161, 162–63,
  169, 170
Carey, E.G., 40
Carter, Jimmy, 5, 128
Center for Health, Environment &
  Justice (CHEJ), 125
Center for Public Environmental
  Oversight (CPEO), 125
Chappell, Marget, 164–65
Cheaper by the Dozen (Gilbreth and
  Carey), 40
Chemical Waste Management, Inc.,
  126
Child welfare agencies (CWA), 101–14
Citizen discontent
  administrative response, 9–14
    accountability, 12, 13
    citizen involvement, 10–14
    collaborative public management,
      12
    informed decision making, 9–10,
      13–14
    managerialism, 12–13
    new public management, 12
    1990s, 11
    1960s–1970s, 10–11
    political economy, 10
    Progressive era, 9–10
    public hearings, 10, 11–12
    reinventing government, 12–13
    transparency, 12
  antigovernment movements, 5, 13
  bureaucrats, 5
  government mistrust, 3–5, 14n1
  historical context
    active citizenship, 6
    constitutional government, 5–6
    eighteenth century, 5–6
    nineteenth century, 6
    pluralistic democracy/politics, 6–7
    populist era, 6
    tax revolts, 7

Citizen discontent
  historical context *(continued)*
    twentieth century, 6–7
    twenty-first century, 7
  justification for
    government power, 7–8
    political economy, 8
    public policy, 8–9
    taxpaying consumers, 8, 9
  outlaw citizenship, 11, 13
  political parties, 5
  politicians, 5
  politics/administration dichotomy, 4
  public opinion, 3–4, 9–10
Citizen involvement dilemmas, 23–25
  citizenship practice, 23–24
  collaborative citizenship, 23–24
  democratic administration, 24–25
  participation defined, 23
Citizen involvement possibilities,
  18–23
  academic responsibility, 21
  administrator facilitation, 22–23
  citizen-centered governance,
    17–18
  citizen complaints, 22
  democratic participation, 20–21
  first wave, 17
  managerialism, 17–18
  Master of Public Administration
    (MPA) survey, 18–23
  new public management, 17–18
  nonprofit organizations, 18
  participation barriers, 20, 21–22
  participation defined, 18, 19
  participation importance, 20–21
  second wave, 17
  third wave, 17–18
"Citizen Participation in Decision
  Making" (Irvin and Stansbury),
  66–67
Citizen participation models
  active model, 86, 91 (table), 93
    (table)
  America*Speaks*, 86, 95–97

Citizen participation models *(continued)*
  collaborative network paradigm, 90, 93 (table)
  effective community governance (ECG), 86, 97–99
  hybrid model, 86, 90, 91 (table)
  ladder of citizen participation, 88, 89 (figure)
  participation defined, 87–88
  passive model, 86, 91 (table), 93 (table)
  public administration, 86–87
  Scorecard of Citizen Participation Methods, 86, 90, 91–100
  state energy policy
    Indiana, 88–90, 91 (table)
    Missouri, 88, 90, 91 (table)
    Ohio, 88, 91 (table)
Citizens' Academy (Miami-Dade County, Florida), 151–52, 153
Citizens Clearinghouse for Hazardous Waste, 125
Citizenship
  as practice, 4
  as status, 4
Citizenship public service role, 60
Civic skills, 37–38
Civil rights
  Seattle Office for Civil Rights (SOCR) (Washington), 159–61
  Title VI, Civil Rights Act (1964), 126, 134
Clean Air Act, 122–23
Clean Water Act, 122–23
Climate change
  drinking water supply, 175
  fossil fuel dependency, 186, 187, 197–99, 202, 208, 209
  rising sea levels, 174–75
  sustainability action plan, 199, 200, 201, 202–6, 207–8, 210, 212
  water conservation, 198–99, 202–4
Clinton, Bill, 12, 130, 134
Coates, P.M., 97
Cognitive empathy, 83

Collaboration
  citizen involvement dilemmas, 23–24
  community-based organizations (CBOs), 106–7
  facilitative leadership, 219
  Team Metro (Miami-Dade County, Florida), 151
  U.S. Environmental Protection Agency (EPA), 136, 139
Collaborative network paradigm, 90, 93 (table)
Collaborative problem-solving, 125, 127, 134
Collaborative public management, 12
Community-based organizations (CBOs)
  administrator responsibility, 113–14
  collaboratives, 106–7
  community alliance, 107–10
  community connection, 105–7
  democratic knowledge, 110–12
  Family to Family (F2F), 103–14
  research background, 103–5
Community engagement
  environmental sustainability narrative, 188, 189–90, 197–99, 200, 201–4, 206–12
  Team Metro (Miami–Dade County, Florida), 147–56
Community land trust (CLT), 217–18
Community outreach
  environmental sustainability narrative, 188, 204–6
  Race and Social Justice Initiative (Seattle, Washington), 165–67, 169
  U.S. Environmental Protection Agency (EPA), 129
Community Roundtable (Seattle, Washington), 171
Competitive grant program, 135
Comprehensive Environmental Response, Compensation, and Liability Act (CERCLA), 122–23, 125, 127, 133

232 INDEX

Congressional Black Caucus, 134
Constitutional government, 5–6, 61–62, 63, 67
Contemporary political theory, 46–48
Cost-benefit analysis
  environmental sustainability narrative, 192–93, 198–99, 202, 208–9, 210
  U.S. Environmental Protection Agency (EPA), 123, 124
"Creative Democracy—The Task Before Us"(Dewey), 34–35
Crossroads, Inc., 161
Curious collaborator, 136, 139
Curtin, Debbie, 148, 149, 152, 155

Davis, Michael, 166–67
Deliberative Practitioner, The (Forester), 94
Democratic action, 216
Democratic administration, 24–25
Democratic governance, 103, 105
Democratic knowledge, 110–12
Democratic living
  administrative challenges, 31–34
  democratic capacity requirements, 36–38
  democratic habits, 35, 36, 38–39
  democratic practices, 35–36, 39–50
    family context, 40–42, 48, 49, 52n2
    school environment, 43–46
    spillover effects, 39–40, 48–50
    workplace, 46–50, 53n7
  fundamental assumptions, 34–36
  research implications, 50–52
Democratic participation, 20–21
Democratic representative accountability feedback loop, 32
Democratic self-governance, 61, 63–65
Dewey, John, 34–35, 64
Disaster recovery
  disaster preparedness, 81, 84
  disaster-resilient community, 81
  disaster-resistance community, 81

Disaster recovery *(continued)*
  empathy, 79–82, 84
  Hurricane Andrew (1992), 147–49
  Hurricane Camille (1969), 80
  Hurricane Isabel (2003), 79, 81
  Hurricane Katrina (2005), 79, 80–82
  Team Metro (Miami–Dade County, Florida), 147–49, 150
  Tropical Storm Danielle (1992), 80
Discipline, 43–45
Downsizing, 13
Drinking water supply, 175

Earth-Cat, 183
Earth Day (1970), 121
Earth Summit (Rio de Janeiro, 1992), 174
Economic development, 188, 190
Economic equity, 160
Economic Opportunity Act (1964), 17
Economic rationality, 65–67
Eco-Village, 166, 167
Educational democratic practices, 43–46
Effective community governance (ECG), 86, 97–99
  model illustration, 98 (figure)
Efficient self-governance, 61, 65–67
Elite self-governance, 61–63
Emergency Planning and Community Right-to-Know Act (EPCRA) (1986), 135
Emotional intelligence, 78
Empathy
  acts of kindness, 82–83
  affective empathy, 83
  AIDS patients, 78–79
  barn raising, 82
  cognitive empathy, 83
  disaster recovery, 79–82, 84
  homelessness, 79
  individualism, 77, 79–81, 82
  micrology, 76
  mirroring behavior, 78–79, 82–83, 84
  personal narrative, 76–78, 82

INDEX 233

Empathy *(continued)*
  public administration correlation,
    83–84
  violent criminals, 79
Energy policy
  energy consumption, 198–99
  fossil fuel dependency, 186, 187,
    197–99, 202, 208, 209
  Indiana, 88–90, 91 (table)
  Missouri, 88, 90, 91 (table)
  Ohio, 68, 88, 91 (table)
Energy Policy Office (Missouri), 91
Environmental Equity (EPA), 134
Environmental Justice Network in
  Action, 166
Environmental Justice and Service
  Equity (Seattle, Washington), 170
Environmental protection. *See* U.S.
  Environmental Protection Agency
  (EPA)
Environmental stewardship
  environmental sustainability
    narrative, 186, 196–97, 202, 209
  U.S. Environmental Protection
    Agency (EPA), 121, 140–42, 143
Environmental sustainability narrative
  administrative meetings, 185–89,
    200–204, 207–12
  communication channels, 188
  community engagement, 188,
    189–90, 197–99, 200, 201–4,
    206–12
  community outreach, 188, 204–6
  environmental stewardship, 186,
    196–97, 202, 209
  green initiatives, 199, 210
  local business engagement, 188, 189,
    193, 197–99, 200, 204–6
  local economic development, 188,
    190
  local employment, 199
  local politics, 187–88, 200–201
  mass transit, 197–98
  media response, 204–6
  public meetings, 188, 189–90, 195

Environmental sustainability narrative
  (continued)
  residential development, 198
  special interest groups, 194
  sustainability action plan
    action items, 193–99, 201–4, 210
    climate change, 199, 200, 201,
      202–6, 207–8, 210, 212
    cost-benefit analysis, 192–93,
      198–99, 202, 208–9, 210
    endorsement for, 206–12
    energy consumption, 198–99
    establishment of, 186–89
    fossil fuel dependency, 186, 187,
      197–99, 202, 208, 209
    opponents, 201, 203, 204, 205–6,
      207–12
    water conservation, 198–99, 202–4
  sustainability coordinator, 186–89
  sustainability task force, 186–90
    Green Team, 196–97, 212
    guiding matrix, 191–92, 193–94,
      196
    guiding principles, 190–91
    meetings, 190–95
    membership, 189–90, 195
    Sounding Board meetings, 192,
      200
    systems thinking, 191–92
    transparency, 202
    work groups, 190, 193–95, 196
Environmental sustainability (Olympia,
  Washington)
  climate change impact
    drinking water supply, 175
    rising sea levels, 174–75
  climate change response
    green initiatives, 175
    public fear, 175
    Sustainability Super Team, 176
    transformational public
      administration, 175–76
Epstein, P., 97
Executive Order 12898, 134
Extra-formal democracy, 24–25

234   INDEX

Facilitative leadership
  citizen representation, 216, 219
  collaboration, 219
  community land trust (CLT), 217–18
  defined, 216
  democratic action, 216
  level playing field, 219
  mass transit example, 221–22
  organizational/institutional change, 221
  participation methods, 220
  portal approach, 221
  relationship improvement, 219
  social movements, 221
  technology, 219–20
  working together, 220–21
Family democratic practices, 40–42, 52n2
Family to Family (F2F)
  administrator responsibility, 112–13
  community-based organization (CBO), 103–14
  community connection, 105–7
  democratic knowledge, 110–12
  public service administration, 108–10, 113–14
  research background, 103–5
  team decision meeting (TDM), 111–12, 113
Federal Emergency Management Agency (FEMA), 81
  Operation Blue Roof, 150
  Project Impact, 81
Federalist Papers, The, 12–13, 17
Federalists, 61–62, 63, 67
Fish Contamination Education Collaborative (FCEC), 127
Flynn, Darlene, 162, 163
Follett, Mary Parker, 64, 94
Forester, J., 94
Fossil fuel dependency, 186, 187, 197–99, 202, 208, 209

Gaebler, T., 12
Gibbs, Lois, 125

Gilbreth, F.B., Jr., 40
Government Information Center (Miami-Dade County, Florida), 147, 156
Government mistrust
  child welfare agencies (CWA), 101–2, 105–6
  citizen discontent, 3–5, 14n1
Government power, 7–8
Government waste, 12–13
Grassroots politics, 87
Great Depression, 10, 68
Great Society, 10
Green initiatives
  environmental sustainability narrative, 196–97, 199, 210, 212
  sustainability (Olympia, Washington), 175
Greenversations, 136

Hamilton, Alexander, 12–13
Harrell, Bruce, 171
Heal the Bay, 127
Historical context
  constitutional government, 5–6, 61–62, 63, 67
  eighteenth century, 5–6
  Federalists, 61–62, 63, 67
  1990s, 11
  1960s–1970s, 10–11
  nineteenth century, 6
  Populist era, 6
  Progressive era, 9–10, 40, 44, 68, 102, 215
  twentieth century, 6–7
  twenty-first century, 7
Homelessness, 79, 170
Hull House (Chicago), 107
Hurricane Andrew (1992), 147–49
Hurricane Camille (1969), 80
Hurricane Isabel (2003), 79, 81
Hurricane Katrina (2005), 79, 80–82
Hybrid participation model
  model characteristics, 91 (table)
  model expansion, 86, 90, 93 (table)

Imagining alternative futures, 61,
71–74
Imagining possibilities, 215–222
Imagining private lives, 61, 70–71,
73–74
*Implementing Citizen Participation in
a Bureaucratic Society* (Kweit and
Kweit), 17
Inclusive Outreach and Public
Engagement Toolkit (Seattle,
Washington), 169
Indiana, 88–90, 91 (table)
Individualism, 77, 79–81, 82
Information technology, 123–24,
135–36, 139
Informed decision making, 9–10,
13–14
Initiative 200 (Washington), 164
Institutional public service role, 60
Institutional racism. *See* Race and
Social Justice Initiative (Seattle,
Washington)
Integrated Federal Interagency
Environmental Justice Action
Agenda, 134
International Association of Public
Participation
Core Values for the Practice of Public
Participation, 132
Spectrum of Participation, 141, 142
(figure)
Internet Web sites
America*Speaks*, 24, 95
Fish Contamination Education
Collaborative (FCEC), 127
Greenversations, 136
Lower Manhattan Development
Corporation (New York City),
97
Regional Plan Association (New York
City), 97
Intrapersonal skills, 37–38, 48
Iowa Citizen-Initiated Performance
Assessment Project, 99
Irvin, R.A., 66–67

Jackson, Andrew, 6, 17
Jackson, Lisa, 132, 143
Jacksonville Community Council, Inc.,
99
Jefferson, Thomas, 64
Johnson, Lyndon, 6–7, 17

Kansas City Metropolitan Energy
Center (Missouri), 90
Keynesian economics, 10
Kweit, M., 17
Kweit, R., 17

Ladder of citizen participation, 88, 89
(figure)
"Ladder of Citizen Participation, A"
(Arnstein), 17
Leavitt, Michael, 132
Libeskind, Daniel, 97
Lobbying, 87
Love Canal (New York), 125
Lower Manhattan Development
Corporation (New York City), 92,
96–97

Madison, James, 17
Managerialism
administrative response, 12–13
citizen involvement possibilities, 17–18
Market-based public service, 12
Mass transit, 197–98, 221–22
Master of Public Administration (MPA)
survey, 18–23
McGinn, Mike, 172
Media, 204–6
Micrology, 76
Mirroring behavior, 78–79, 82–83, 84
Missouri, 88, 90, 91 (table)
*Model Plan for Public Participation,
The* (NEJAC), 131–32
Moral education, 43–44
Moral theory, 78

National Academy of Public
Administration, 135

236 INDEX

National Advisory Council for Environmental Policy and Technology (NACEPT), 121, 142, 144n2
National Association of Counties (NACo) Achievement Awards, 151
National Environmental Justice Advisory Council (NEJAC), 124, 131–32, 135
Native Americans, 130–31
Natural disasters. *See* Disaster recovery
Neighborhood Matching Grant (Seattle, Washington), 170
Neighborhood organizations, 64, 68–69
Neighborhood PRIDE (Miami-Dade County, Florida), 151, 152
Neoliberalism, 65–67
Network governance, 12
Neuroscience, 78–79, 82–83, 84
New public management
 administrative response, 12
 citizen involvement possibilities, 17–18
 efficiency perspective, 65–67
New Public Service, 102–3
New State, The (Follett), 94
Nickels, Greg, 159, 171
NIMBY (Not In My Backyard), 25, 95, 99–100
Nixon, Richard, 121
Nonprofit organizations, 18
Nonprofit partnerships
 accountability, 101, 112
 active citizenship, 102–3, 105
 administrator responsibility, 112–13
 advocacy, 106–10
 child welfare agency (CWA), 101–14
 community connection, 105–7
 democratic governance, 103, 105
 democratic knowledge, 110–12
 Family to Family (F2F), 103–14
 New Public Service, 102–3
 public service administration, 107–10
 research background, 103–5

Nonprofit partnerships *(continued)*
 research implications, 113–14
 settlement house movement, 101, 102, 107–10

Obama, Barack, 3, 11, 78, 143
Office of Energy Development (Indiana), 91
Office of Neighborhood Compliance (Miami–Dade County, Florida), 147, 153, 156
Ohio, 68, 88, 91 (table)
Ohio Energy Office, 91
Operation Blue Roof (FEMA), 150
Oregon, 68
Osborne, D., 12
Outlaw citizenship, 11, 13

Palos Verdes Shelf (California), 127
Participation and Democratic Theory (Pateman), 46–47
Passive participation model
 model characteristics, 91 (table)
 model expansion, 86, 93 (table)
Pataki, George, 92
Pateman, C., 46–47
Patriarchal structure, 40–42, 49
Peacock, Marcus, 136
People's Institute, The, 161
Performance audits, 12
Pew Research Center for the People and the Press, 3–4
Political capacity, 37–38
Political economy, 8, 10
Political knowledge, 37–38
Political parties, 5
Politicians, 5
Politics
 astroturf-roots politics, 87
 Congressional Black Caucus, 134
 contemporary political theory, 46–48
 environmental sustainability narrative, 187–88, 200–201
 grassroots politics, 87
 pluralistic democracy/politics, 6–7

Politics *(continued)*
Race and Social Justice Initiative
(Seattle, Washington), 171–72
Team Metro (Miami-Dade County,
Florida), 152–53, 154
Politics/administration dichotomy, 4
Populist era, 6
Prince William County, Virginia,
Governing for Results Cycles, 99
Privatization, 13
Progressive era, 9–10, 40, 44, 68, 102,
215
Project CHART (Miami–Dade County,
Florida), 148
Project Impact (FEMA), 81
Proposition 13 (California), 7
Public Administration Review, 66–67
Public Broadcasting System (PBS), 162
Public hearings
citizen discontent, 10, 11–12
environmental sustainability
narrative, 188, 189–90, 195
*Public Knowledge and Perceptions
of Chemical Risks in Six
Communities* (EPA), 137
Public opinion, 3–4, 9–10
*Public Participation in Public
Decisions* (Thomas), 92, 94
Public service techniques
citizen involvement
contemporary status, 69
historical context, 67–69
citizen self-governance
Athenians model, 63–64
contemporary context, 63, 64–67
democratic perspective, 61, 63–65
economic rationality, 65–67
efficiency perspective, 61, 65–67
elite perspective, 61–63
historical context, 61–64
neighborhood organizations, 64,
68–69
imagining alternative futures, 61,
71–74
imagining possibilities, 215–222

Public service techniques *(continued)*
imagining private lives, 61, 70–71,
73–74
public employee role, 59–61
administrative discretion, 59
citizenship public service role, 60
contributory perspective, 59–60
institutional public service role, 60
neutrality perspective, 59–60
research implications, 73–74
See also Facilitative leadership

Race and Social Justice Initiative
(Seattle, Washington)
assessment of
organizational structure, 173
relationships and deliverables,
172–73
shared vision, 172, 173
capacity building, 160, 161, 162–63,
169, 170
city demographics, 157, 167–68
citywide accomplishments
administrative operations, 170
Budget and Policy Filter, 169
capacity building, 170
contracting equity, 169–70
outreach and public engagement
policy, 169
Racial Equity Toolkit, 169, 172
translation and interpretation
policy, 169
workforce equity, 170
community outreach, 165–67, 169
community profile, 157–59
Community Roundtable, 171
contracting equity, 163–65, 169–70
coordinating teams, 160–61, 163,
169, 172
core teams, 160–61
departmental work plans, 160
economic equity, 160
Environmental Justice and Service
Equity, 170
guiding principles, 159–60, 170–71

238   INDEX

Race and Social Justice Initiative
    (Seattle, Washington) *(continued)*
    historically underutilized businesses
        (HUB), 163–65
    immigrant/refugee services, 160, 169
    implementation, 158–59
    Inclusive Outreach and Public
        Engagement Toolkit, 169
    institutional racism, 158–59
    Neighborhood Matching Grant, 170
    organizational structure, 160–61
    political opportunities, 171–72
    public engagement, 160
    Seattle Office for Civil Rights
        (SOCR), 159–61
    Seattle Public Utilities (SPU),
        161–68
        community outreach, 165–67
        employee training, 162–63
        minority contracts, 163–65
        service equity, 167–68
    Ten-Year Plan to End Homelessness,
        170
    women and minority business
        enterprises (WMBE), 163–64
    workforce equity, 160, 170
Race—The Power of an Illusion (PBS),
    162
Racial Equity Toolkit (Seattle,
    Washington), 169, 172
Reagan, Ronald, 5, 12, 67, 68, 129
Reinventing government movement,
    12–13
Reinventing Government (Osborne and
    Gaebler), 12
Resource Conservation and Recovery
    Act, 122–23, 124–25, 133
Results that Matter (Epstein, Coates,
    and Wray), 97
Roosevelt, Franklin D., 10
Ruckelshaus, William, 122, 129

San Jose Department of Streets and
    Traffic, 99
Schlozman, K.L., 39

Scientific knowledge, 9–10
Scientific management, 12–13, 40, 107,
    110
Scorecard of Citizen Participation
    Methods
    active participation model, 93 (table)
    America*Speaks*
        "Listen to the City" (New York),
            24, 95, 96–97
        Washington, DC, Citizen Summits,
            95–96
    collaborative network paradigm, 93
        (table)
    effective community governance
        (ECG), 86, 97–99
    model expansion, 86, 90, 91–100
    participation evaluation, 99–100
    passive participation model, 93
        (table)
Sea levels, 174–75
Seattle Office for Civil Rights (SOCR)
    (Washington), 159–61
Seattle Process (Washington), 165–66
Seattle Public Utilities (SPU)
    (Washington), 161–68
Settlement house movement, 101, 102,
    107–10
    administrative hierarchy, 107,
        108–9
    gendered roles, 107
    scientific management, 107, 110
Shintech (Louisiana), 126
Smith, Darryl, 172
Social capacity, 35
Social capitalism, 40
Social networks, 35
Socioeconomic status (SES), 42, 46
Special needs transportation
    (Washington), 221–22
St. Anslem's, 127
Stansbury, J., 66–67
Stierheim, Merrett, 152
Stivers, C., 107
"Study of Administration, The"
    (Wilson), 9, 62–63

INDEX 239

Superfund. *See* Comprehensive Environmental Response, Compensation, and Liability Act (CERCLA)
Sustainability (Olympia, Washington)
climate change impact
drinking water supply, 175
rising sea levels, 174–75
climate change response
green initiatives, 175
public fear, 175
Sustainability Super Team, 176
transformational public administration, 175–76
community profile, 174–75
Department of Public Works (DPW)
creativity and passion, 181–82
decision-making tools, 177–81
delegation, 182
departmental reorganization, 176–77
human resource systems, 181
organizational structure, 181–83
purpose-centered leadership, 182–83
siloed operational structure, 176
Sustainable Action Map (SAM), 177–81
Evergreen State College, The 174, 177
McAllister Springs, 175
sustainability barriers
administrative response, 176–83
balanced decision making, 176
citizen inspiration, 176
defining sustainability, 176
transformative strategies, 183–84
Sustainable Action Map (SAM), 177–81
illustration, 178 (figure)
key dimensions, 177–78
NICE components, 177
potential uses, 180
processes of, 178–80
Stoplight system, 178, 179–80
SWOT analysis, 177–78, 179
Systems thinking, 191–92

Targeted Community Initiative (Orange County, Florida), 217–18
Taxpaying consumers, 8, 9
Tax revolts, 7
Taylor, Frederick, 12–13, 40
Team decision meeting (TDM), 111–12, 113
Team Metro (Miami-Dade County, Florida)
agency creation, 148
agency demise, 147, 150, 152–55
agency evolution, 147–56
community engagement, 147–56
assessment of, 155
Citizens' Academy, 151–52, 153
collaboration, 151
Neighborhood PRIDE, 151, 152
transparency, 151, 153, 155, 156
disaster recovery, 147–49, 150
funding, 152–53, 154, 156
Government Information Center (GIC), 147, 156
Office of Neighborhood Compliance (ONC), 147, 153, 156
politics, 152–53, 154
Project CHART, 148
Team Metro South Dade Office, 148
Technical assistance grant (TAG), 133
Technocrats, 6, 10
Technology
facilitative leadership, 219–20
U.S. Environmental Protection Agency (EPA), 123–24, 135–36, 139
Ten-Year Plan to End Homelessness (Seattle, Washington), 170
Thatcher, Margaret, 12
Thomas, J.C., 92, 94
Title VI, Civil Rights Act (1964), 126, 134
Toxic Substances Control Act, 122–23
Train, Russell, 122
Transparency
citizen discontent, 12, 18–19

240   INDEX

Transparency *(continued)*
environmental protection, 129, 132,
    143
environmental sustainability
    narrative, 202
Team Metro (Miami-Dade County,
    Florida), 151, 153, 155, 156
Transportation, 197–98, 221–22
Tropical Storm Danielle (1992), 80

University of Michigan, 3
U.S. Environmental Protection Agency
    (EPA)
Community Action for a Renewed
    Environment (CARE), 135
Conflict Prevention and Resolution
    Center, 131
environmental protection
    cost-benefit analysis, 123, 124
    environmental impact analysis,
        123–25
    environmental permits, 124–25,
        126
    legislative policy, 122–23, 132–35
    risk assessment models, 123–24
Final Report of the Federal Facilities
    Environmental Restoration and
    Dialogue Committee (1996),
    134–35
Framework for Cumulative Risk
    Assessment, 124
Interagency Working Group (IWG),
    133, 144n5
Office of Children's Health
    Protection, 131
Office of Community and
    Intergovernmental Liaison, 130
Office of Environmental Education,
    130
Office of Environmental Equity, 130,
    134
Office of Environmental Justice, 130
Office of Intergovernmental
    Relations, 129–30
Office of Press Services, 128

U.S. Environmental Protection Agency
    (EPA) *(continued)*
Office of the Administrator, 131
Office of the Ombudsman, 133
Office of Public Affairs, 128, 129,
    130
Office of Public and Private Liaison,
    129–30
Office of Public Awareness, 128
Office of Water, 131
organizational development, 128–42
    agency evolution, 121–26
    authoritative role, 137
    convener role, 138–39
    curious collaborator, 136, 139
    evolving roles, 121–22, 136–42
    federal departments, 128–35
    neutral arbiter role, 138
    stewardship role, 121, 140–42,
        143
policy development, 128–42
    competitive grant program, 135
    statutory/program mandates,
        122–23, 132–35, 140–41
    technical assistance grant (TAG),
        133
    technology impact, 123–24,
        135–36, 139
    toxic pollution, 135
    transparency, 129, 132, 143
    waste-management, 133–35
public health impacts, 123–25
public interaction, 120–21, 143
    activism, 126
    assimilation, 129
    civil rights, 126, 134
    collaborative problem-solving,
        125, 127, 134
    community-based organizations
        (CBOs), 125–26, 127
    dialogue, 129
    environmental justice movement,
        124, 127, 133–35
    feedback, 129
    group identification, 129

INDEX 241

U.S. Environmental Protection Agency
(EPA)
public interaction *(continued)*
outreach, 129
policy development, 128–42
public trust, 122, 124
Spectrum of Participation, 141,
142 (figure)
Public Involvement Policy, 132
Right to Know, 135
Toxic Release Inventory (TRI), 135
"Transparency in EPA's Operations,"
132, 143
Tribal Office, 130–31
U.S. Forest Service, 18

Verba, S., 39
Violent criminals, 79
Voice and Equality (Verba, Schlozman,
and Brady), 39

Ward-republic, 64
War on Poverty, 7, 17
Washington
Initiative 200, 164
neighborhood organizations, 68–69

Washington *(continued)*
Seattle Office for Civil Rights
(SOCR), 159–61
Seattle Public Utilities (SPU),
161–68
See also Race and Social Justice
Initiative (Seattle, Washington);
Sustainability (Olympia,
Washington)
Waste-management policy, 133–35
Waste Technologies Industries (Ohio),
126
Water supply
conservation efforts, 198–99, 202–4
drinking water, 175
legislation, 122–23
Western States Center, 161
Williams, Anthony, 95–96
Wilson, Woodrow, 9, 62–63
Workplace democratic practices,
46–50, 53n7
World Trade Center (New York), 24,
91–92, 96–97
World War I, 68
World War II, 68
Wray, L.D., 97

CPSIA information can be obtained
at www.ICGtesting.com
Printed in the USA
BVHW04s0525010918
525902BV00018B/62/P